The TRAUMA
TREATMENT
HANDBOOK

The TRAUMA TREATMENT HANDBOOK

Protocols Across the Spectrum

ROBIN SHAPIRO

Foreword by Daniel J. Siegel

W. W. Norton & Company
New York · London

For information about special discounts for bulk purchases, please contact
W. W. Norton
Special Sales at specialsales@wwnorton.com or 800-233-4830

Manufacturing by R. R. Donnelly, Bloomsburg
Book design by Charlotte Staub
Production manager: Leeann Graham

Library of Congress Cataloging-in-Publication Data

Shapiro, Robin.
  The trauma treatment handbook : protocols across the spectrum / Robin Shapiro ;
foreword by Daniel J. Siegel. — 1st ed.
     p. ; cm.
  "A Norton professional book."
  Includes bibliographical references and index.
  ISBN 978-0-393-70618-5 (hardcover)
  1. Post-traumatic stress disorder—Treatment.   2. Psychic trauma.   I. Title.
  [DNLM: 1. Stress Disorders, Post-Traumatic—therapy.   2. Psychotherapy—
methods.   3. Stress Disorders, Post-Traumatic—psychology.   WM 172 S525t
2010]
  RC552.P67S45 2010
  616.85'21—dc22   2010013117

ISBN: 978-0-393-70618-5

W. W. Norton & Company, Inc., 500 Fifth Avenue, New York, N.Y. 10110
www.wwnorton.com
W. W. Norton & Company Ltd., Castle House, 75/76 Wells Street,
London W1T 3QT

3   4   5   6   7   8   9   0

*Dedicated to the memory of my mentor, Thom Negri,
and to all the past and present clinicians, innovators,
teachers, and clients who have taught me to heal trauma.*

CONTENTS

ACKNOWLEDGMENTS

I didn't write this book alone. Thank you to all the people who helped me directly. The obvious ones are:

Kathy Steele, who, seemingly patiently, set me straight about many aspects of structural dissociation. For anything that is correct about SD, I give her credit. For anything that isn't, please blame me.

David Calof, my long-time consultant, who provided much of the structure and information for the clinical hypnosis chapter.

David Kearney, a physician who told me about his yoga and mindfulness training program at the Seattle VA.

Martha Jacobi, who let me crib from her prepublished descriptions of two kinds of somatic therapies.

Diana Fosha, who allowed me to steal liberally from a section of her book about psychodynamic therapies.

Sharon Stanley, who explained somatic transformation to me.

Marcia Herival, who vetted the exposure and CBT chapters and gave me more modalities to research.

Wayne McClesky, who reviewed the energy psychology chapter (years after teaching me most of what I know about it).

Jim Cole, who did the same for the reenactment protocol, the only intervention I know that ends with a giggle.

Trisha Pearce, who filled me in about working with military and veterans during a 40-minute phone call and had already trained me through her wonderful volunteer Soldiers Project NW.

Thank you to all the other teachers, trainers, authors, and consultants who taught me so much about trauma and its treatments. I hope I did you justice and that I got the references right.

Thank you, in advance, to each of you who are choosing to heal trauma as your life's work.

Thanks to the people at Norton Professional Books who suggested I write this book and urged me to keep it user-friendly. Thank you to Andrea Costella, Kristen Holt-Browning, and Vani Kannan for guiding me, once again, through the publishing process. I tried to get it write, I mean, right, the first time.

Thank you, one more time, to my first reader and first editor, my mother, writer Elly Welt. I continue to improve my writing under your tutelage. Yes, I got the message about italics and quotation marks.

And to my long-suffering husband, Doug Plummer, who supported me in all ways through yet another book, including providing two more wonderful photos: I adore you.

ACRONYMS

AB/ISTDP: attachment-based intensive short-term dynamic psycho-therapy

ACT: acceptance and commitment therapy; accept, choose, take action

AEDP: accelerated experiential-dynamic psychotherapy

AET: accelerated empathetic therapy

ANP: apparently normal part (in structural dissociation)

APA: American Psychological Association

ASD: acute stress disorder

BLS: bilateral stimulation (in EMDR)

BPD: borderline personality disorder

BSP: Brainspotting

CBT: cognitive behavior therapy

COS: combat operational stress

CPT: cognitive processing therapy

CT: cognitive therapy

CTSD: complex traumatic stress disorders

DBT: dialectical behavior therapy

DDIS: Dissociative Disorders Interview Scale

DDNOS: dissociative disorder not otherwise specified

DDP: dyadic developmental psychotherapy

DES: Dissociative Experiences Scale

DESNOS: disorders of extreme stress, not otherwise specified

DID: dissociative identity disorder (formerly multiple personality disorder, MPD)

DNMS: developmental needs-meeting strategy

DSM-IV: Diagnostic and Statistical Manual of Mental Disorders

DTD: developmental trauma disorder

EFT: emotional freedom technique

EMDR: eye movement desensitization and reprocessing

EP: emotional part (in structural dissociation)

EX: exposure therapy

HSP: highly sensitive person

IFS: internal family systems

ISSTD: International Society for the Study of Trauma and Dissociation

ISTDP: intensive short-term dynamic psychotherapy

LENS: low-energy neurofeedback system

MBSR: mindfulness-based stress reduction

NAS: nurturing adult self (in DNMS)

PAS: protective adult self (in DNMS)

PE: prolonged exposure

PTP: pretraumatized person (in the structural dissociation model)

PTSD: posttraumatic stress disorder

REBT: rational emotive behavior therapy

RP: reenactment protocol

SCS: Spiritual Core Self (in DNMS)

SD: structural dissociation

SDM: strategic developmental model

SDQ: Somatoform Disorder Questionnaire

SE: somatic experiencing

SIDS: sudden infant death syndrome

SIT: stress inoculation therapy

SP: sensorimotor psychotherapy

SSRI: selective serotonin reuptake inhibitor

STDP: short-term dynamic psychotherapy

TBI: traumatic brain injury

TFT: thought field therapy

WTF?: response to so many acronyms!

FOREWORD

Trauma is an experience that overwhelms our ability to cope and leaves our relationships and our brains with the challenge of finding a way to remain integrated and functioning well. In many ways, a psychotherapist working with individuals who have been traumatized needs to use the trusting therapeutic relationship to cultivate healing by attuning to the internal world of the client and resonating with that experience. Robin Shapiro has written a practical guide to a wide range of treatment strategies for trauma that offer useful approaches to tracking and transforming traumatic symptoms and guiding the individual toward healing.

Healing—becoming whole—can be seen as a process of integration, linking the internal neural circuits that have become disconnected during the overwhelming events in a person's life. For therapists, staying present with trauma is not easy, and having a wide range of creative steps easily accessible in the clinicians' "tool kit" makes the process more likely to be effective. The journey to learn a broad range of treatment approaches included in this book has enabled Shapiro to offer her clinical wisdom; she demonstrates in clear summaries and helpful clinical vignettes how to apply these specific techniques in particular clinical situations.

All psychotherapy needs to be individually tailored to the person presenting for treatment. In this way, we as therapists need to have a spectrum of interventions at our disposal in order to create the most effective and individually sculpted therapeutic experiences. When I first skimmed over this handbook, I thought that the lack of scientific studies supporting many of the various individual approaches would lead me to call the author and say that I could not write this foreword. But as I read each chapter and reflected on my own development as a therapist, I realized that this compilation was indeed a very helpful compendium of useful—even if mostly not scientifically proven—approaches that would help any clinician working with traumatized individuals. These are the tools of the art of psychotherapy. So I read on and found myself soaking in the author's sensitivity, her directness, her compassionate reflections on the therapeutic process, and her skill at extracting the best from a range of clinical strategies to help the healing process evolve and be more likely to find a window of opportunity to make lasting change possible.

It takes an open mind and much time and energy to learn each of the different approaches and specific techniques included in this book. What this book offers is the rich clinical experience of a range of interventions all within one text. Are they each scientifically proven to work? No. Will they be helpful to every single patient? Unlikely. But as each person is different, and each person's trauma unique, so, too, does the treatment approach for every person require a special creative configuration assembled by a well-prepared, sensitive, and open-minded clinician.

This book is a wonderful offering from a caring and well-educated therapist's wise and thoughtful integration of a range of approaches. Clinicians in training and those with years of experience who read this work will find themselves enriched by the author's broad knowledge and clinical expertise. And those traumatized people who are fortunate enough to be treated by therapists who have read this work and benefited from Shapiro's hard and loving synthesis will be all the better for their efforts. Read on and take in the applied knowledge of the collective efforts to heal trauma at its core.

— Daniel J. Siegel, MD

The TRAUMA
TREATMENT
HANDBOOK

INTRODUCTION

As psychotherapists, we are privileged to use our whole selves to help our clients heal from traumatic wounds. While connecting deeply with them, we use our detective brains to puzzle out what is happening with them and what to do about it. We enjoy helping single-trauma survivors quickly get back to their lives. We combine a variety of techniques to slowly and carefully help our most dissociative clients transform into their integrated selves. We are lucky to learn new skills from the innovators in our field and in creative collaboration with our clients. We are privileged to hang out with colleagues who love their work and support ours. Throughout each therapy we are delighted to hear, "I finally know it's over!" "I feel like 'me' again!" "It wasn't my fault. I was a little kid when that happened." "I've got my body back!" "I can have sex again." "I didn't have one nightmare all week!" "Thank you for letting me get completely here and now!" "I've got my life back!"

My colleague Deborah Woolley says it well: "I am drawn to trauma therapy because it offers me an opportunity to do something about the brokenness all around us. Doing this work is an experience of confronting that brokenness head-on and in its place restoring wholeness" (personal communication, November 2009).

There is no one perfect trauma therapy. True believers think there is and that clients whom they cannot heal with their favored modality are either resistant or hopeless cases. There is a broader way of thinking. You can learn many trauma therapies, see clients through diverse theoretical lenses, and synthesize aspects of many modalities into your work. This book cannot teach you how to do most of the therapies, since almost all of them are too complex for this format. It will give you resources—the books, Web sites, and articles—from which you can pursue training.

ORDER

The first two chapters describe the effects of trauma and the array of trauma diagnoses. Because the *Diagnostic and Statistical Manual (DSM-IV)* definitions are incomplete, I add descriptions that fit the newest research (Courtois & Ford, 2009; van der Kolk, 1996). The next two chapters discuss assessment and client preparation. The middle of the book describes trauma therapies that may be used for simple trauma. The following section deals with therapies for complex trauma and dissociation. There is a brief unit about specific client populations: survivors of war, sexual assault, traumatic grief, and relational trauma. The last chapter is about how to take care of yourself while doing this work.

When you read about the trauma therapies, look for these five threads, which may be implicit or explicit, in each modality:

1. *Presence*: Getting into the here-and-now experience of body, affect, and thought. That includes aiding clients to be in the window of tolerance, that is, not overstimulated or overmobilized, not immobilized or shut down, but present and capable of connection so that the work can move through them (Ogden, Minton, & Pain, 2006; Porges, 1995, 2001).

2. *Dual attention*: In good trauma therapy, clients must be in two places at once: they must hold the trauma in mind (exposure), while maintaining focus in the current time and place. In EMDR, the second focus is the bilateral stimulation. In yoga and somatic work, it is attention to bodily experience. In good relational analytic work, the dual attention is the therapeutic relationship that keeps one part of the mind connected in the present and the other in the traumatic past. In ego state work, it's the current self that connects with the distressed younger part.

3. *Affect (emotion) while in relationship*: In trauma work, clients have affective experiences while held inside the window of toler-

ance and a therapeutic relationship. It's not that the affect is discharged, though it might be. It's that it is felt and not avoided, then witnessed and survived, then transformed into a memory and no longer a developmental catastrophe. Myriad studies show that the strength of the therapeutic relationship is the strongest predictor of a good outcome (Lambert & Barley, 2001; Schore, 2009).

4. *Relationship with self and the other*: Clients gain tolerance and acceptance of their own affect and history and the capacity for relating to others.

5. *Making meaning of the traumatic events*: This is the final stage of many trauma therapies (often accompanied by anger, then grief, then great relief).

While you examine each modality, ask yourself these questions:

- How does this therapy see clients or problems?
- What would I do with a particular client using this therapy?
- How must I bend this treatment to accommodate a particular client?
- Is this the best treatment for this client? If not, what therapy or therapies will do the job?
- Are there parts of this modality that dovetail with other work that I already do?

ALPHABET SOUP

Just after the table of contents is a list of every abbreviation and acronym in the book. You won't have to look through the entire book or the index for the first mention of an abbreviation. To find out what ASD or DESNOS or SSRI stands for, go to the acronym pages.

RESEARCH

If you want a comprehensive review of the research literature, read *Effective Treatments for PTSD: Practice Guidelines from the International Society for Traumatic Stress Studies,* by Foa, Keane, and Friedman (2000). Another good resource is the Publications page of Bessel van der Kolk's Web site (http://www.traumacenter.org/

products/publications.php). Research is beyond the scope of most of this book. I mention it when describing alternative therapies: mindfulness, energy psychology, and neurofeedback. Understand that there are battles between proponents of some of the major therapies, using research studies to win their arguments. They tend to look at the research that proves that their modality is best and ignore the valid research that doesn't. I am staying out of the fray. I use phenomenological research. If a therapy makes the symptoms change quickly and permanently, without causing further distress, I'll do it again.

Warning

Throughout the book, I use realistic depictions of different kinds of traumatic experiences. If you have an unresolved trauma history, some vignettes may trigger your own trauma symptoms. Make sure that you stay mindful and take care of yourself while reading the distressing parts. Breathe deeply and keep your feet planted on the floor. Take breaks when necessary. And if you feel terrible after you put the book down, it might be time to seek a good, effective trauma therapist.

Part I

TRAUMA AND DISSOCIATION

CHAPTER ONE

Trauma

trauma: a. an experience that produces psychological injury or pain. b. the psychological injury so caused. (Dictionary.com, 2009)

trauma: An emotional wound or shock that creates substantial, lasting damage to the psychological development of a person, often leading to neurosis. (*American Heritage Dictionary of the English Language*, 2006)

The American Psychiatric Association's (2000) definition of post-traumatic stress disorder (PTSD; see appendix) tells us that PTSD comes after "a life-threatening event" that creates "intense fear, help-lessness, or horror." It goes on to say that these events can include rape, war, car accidents, or cataclysms. People with PTSD suffer in-trusive dreams or visual, cognitive, or physical flashbacks of the event and a sense that it is still happening in the present. They try to avoid anything that reminds them of the trauma. When they are reminded, they can have huge physical and emotional reactions. They may feel numb, or hyperaroused, hopeless, estranged, and not themselves. They may be sleepless, angry, and find it hard to focus. And they may feel that they or the world are doomed. If symptoms happen within a month of the bad event, they are called acute stress disorder (ASD; see appendix). After a month, these symptoms are PTSD.

In my clinical experience, it doesn't take a life-threatening event to create a trauma reaction. Babies can display the biological markers of trauma if their mothers show a still, nonresponsive face (Tronick, 2007). Children or adults may show a trauma response to an angry, yelling parent, boss, or partner, a job loss, or an embarrassing situation. Successful therapy can heal these relational traumas with big changes in affect, behavior, and cognition.

Stephen Porges (1995, 2001, 2005) has an elegant explanation of what trauma does to us. He describes how the vagus nerve runs through the torso up to the brain and has two parts that complement the arousal function of the sympathetic nervous system. The ventral vagus originates in an area toward the front of the brainstem and the dorsal vagus originates in an area toward the back of the brainstem. The dorsal branch is unmyelinated and the ventral branch is myelinated, which enables more minute and rapid neural regulation of the visceral organs. Moreover, the ventral branch is anatomically connected with the areas of the brainstem that control the striated muscles of the face, head, and neck. When the myelinated ventral vagus is engaged, we can eat, connect with other people, and use our big brains to work, create, and be interested in what's around us. When we sense a threat, the unmyelinated ventral vagus puts us into a mobilized state, capable of scanning for danger and defending ourselves. We cannot eat, socially connect, or use much intellectual capacity when we're mobilized. When we think we're going to be killed, or after a too-extended mobilized state, the dorsal vagus turns on and turns down every function that isn't about baseline physical survival: an immobilized state. When we're not being threatened, these three functions of the vagal system constantly and subtly adjust our bodies, including our brains. Momentary, not-too-big distressing experiences can mobilize the system, then fade away as the system readjusts. Stronger, longer, developmentally ill-timed, or repetitive trauma can have long-lasting effects.

BEST-CASE SCENARIO: TRAUMATIC EVENT WITH FEW LASTING EFFECTS

A person with a healthy nervous system responds to danger by mobilizing, discharging, and making sense of the trauma by talking and dreaming, then returning to a normal connected, attentive state.

> The oncoming pickup truck swerves across the line into your lane. In milliseconds your body mobilizes. You fixate on the pickup. Your digestive system shuts down. Your brain narrows its attention to awareness of threat and shuts down the parts that aren't about

responding to danger (hitting the brakes, turning the car, avoiding the other cars). You can't pay attention to your passenger or the radio talking to you, because the muscles in your ears are too tight, reset for low tones only, the sounds of predators (Porges, 1995, 2001). Your heart rate increases. Adrenalin pumps into your bloodstream to enable you to protect yourself. You begin to oxygenate your system so that you can act: fight or flee. You're in total unmyelinated ventral vagal mode.

You steer to the right as the pickup swerves into its own lane, and within minutes your body begins to reset itself. You shake for a moment as the adrenaline starts clearing out. You tell yourself, "I don't believe I survived, but I did." You might go limp and feel spaced out (dorsal vagal response, as your body recuperates from its mobilized state). If you started out with a relatively trauma-free life, good engaged parents, and a stalwart nervous system, you might feel shaky for a half hour to a few days. You find yourself telling the story of your escape to everyone you meet. You might have a few restless nights with weird dreams. And then it's over. Your body resets to its normal social, interested-in-life (myelinated ventral vagal) settings. You get hungry. You can think. You want and are able to connect with people. You get on with life. If something reminds you of the near accident, you might feel a little watchful, but you're fine.

MEDIUM-BAD SCENARIO: TRAUMATIC EVENT, ACUTE STRESS, THEN PTSD

The Trauma

The pickup truck jumps into your lane and hits your car with a bang. The airbag and the window explode in your face as your car flips upside down. You can feel blood dripping from your nose and off the top of your head, and you hear the screaming of a person in the other car. You're stuck. You can't get yourself out and your body reflexively jerks as cars swerve around you. Your heart is beating loudly in your ears. Your body wants to move, but you can't undo the seatbelt without falling. Your brain reacts to every sight and sound, with more waves of panic. You hear sirens and soon the police are asking questions, which you can barely understand. They seem scared, wondering if they can get you out before the car catches fire. Since the threat of death seems imminent, and you can't move, your body enters an immobilized (dorsal vagal) state. You go limp. Your brain gets fuzzy. Your brain pumps its own opiates into your body so that death won't hurt so much. With all those endogenous opiates aboard, it's hard to care that you can't move or think. Your body barely responds when they pull you out and hand you to the EMTs and while you're not unconscious, things feel far away. You hear someone say that your nose is broken, but you can't feel it. The rest of the day in the ambulance and in the emergency room is a blur of concerned faces, poking needles, and waiting.

Acute Stress Disorder

Every night, in your dreams, you relive the crash. You don't want to drive. You especially don't want to drive past that corner. You don't want to do anything that reminds you of the accident. You're irritable about everything. You jump at every unexpected noise. As your amygdala in your primitive brain keeps sending danger signals, you find yourself reliving the event over and over. You hear the brakes squeal, the glass breaking, and the sensation of being suspended upside down, but you can't remember getting out and the ambulance trip. You know it's over, but the part of your brain that is oriented in time and space keeps going offline and you feel like you're in the middle of the accident. Even though you know that it wasn't your fault, you feel guilty and keep trying to figure out what you could have done differently. "I should have noticed that guy in the truck earlier. He would still be alive if I'd gotten out of the way." Sometimes you feel really weird, as if you're floating out of your body (depersonalization) or aren't really yourself (derealization). And when you're not freaked out, guilty, or angry, you're going into a dorsal vagal or shutdown state again and not feeling much of anything. It's as if you don't care about your sweetheart, your friends, your classes or job, and your favorite pastimes. You feel dull and sort of stupid. Sometimes, you feel like you have to sleep, but it's more like passing out, and you don't really feel rested after you wake up. It's hard to work. It's hard to connect. Sometimes you just stay home. You notice that if you have a few drinks, you can get to sleep. You find yourself drinking more.

PTSD

Months have passed, and you get a little better. Sometimes, when you're not in a car, you feel normal. You can do your work, connect a little better with the people in your life, and sometimes even concentrate fully on what you're doing. You feel a broader range of emotions. Sometimes, when you're with friends, or connected to your sweetheart, you feel really good (myelinated ventral vagal/socially engaged state). If anything unexpected happens, especially if you're on the road, your body jumps back into mobilized states. If you even think of the accident, it feels like it's happening again, right now. And sometimes, when you're not even thinking about it, you see that truck speeding toward you again and you feel yourself tensing up and bracing for the crash.

You won't go near the area of the accident. You absolutely don't want to talk about it. You still don't like to drive. It's hard to sleep at night and the crash still haunts your dreams. You alternate between feeling too little and feeling too much, going from feeling numb to startled, angry, or hopeless. The more time passes, the crazier you feel. You start worrying about your family and friends. "What if something happens?" you ask yourself. "What's wrong with me? Shouldn't I be over this by now?" You find yourself turning to alcohol, more and more, and feel shame for still having the flashbacks, the drinking, and the bad moods.

COMPLEX TRAUMATIC STRESS DISORDERS

There is more to trauma than PTSD. Many pathological manifestations of trauma come from non-life-threatening events, including relational trauma, shaming incidents, deprivation, bullying, occupational stress, and body-generated states. A panic attack won't kill you but is almost always traumatic. A public humiliation can be devastating. Breakups or any kind of social abandonment can bring on all the symptoms of PTSD. When these traumas are historically rare, they are often more amenable to treatment than PTSD. When they are pervasive, they can create entrenched many-faceted pathologies: complex traumatic stress disorders (Courtois & Ford, 2009).

Chronic exposure to childhood abuse or neglect can reshape personalities around the pathology of trauma. Researchers and clinicians are developing new diagnoses for these complex traumatic stress disorders. Developmental trauma disorder (DTD) is a diagnosis for children who have the following:

A. Chronic exposure to interpersonal trauma, including abandonment, betrayal, or witnessing or receiving any form of abuse.
B. A triggered pattern of repeated emotional, somatic, behavioral, relational, self-blaming or cognitive dysregulation in response to trauma cues.
C. Persistently altered attributions and expectancies, including distrust, negative self-attribution, lack of recourse or belief in help or justice, and a sense of inevitability of future victimization.
D. Functional impairment in educational, peer, legal, or vocational spheres. (van der Kolk, 2005)

These children are often dissociative (see Chapter 3), too passive, or too unruly and likely to be misdiagnosed with ADHD or insufficiently diagnosed with depression.

Kids with DTD can turn into adults with disorders of extreme stress not otherwise specified (DESNOS; see appendix) (Luxenberg, Spinazzola, & van der Kolk, 2001). DESNOS clients have trouble regulating their emotions. They may be angry, suicidal, and either obsequious or engaging in risky or self-destructive behaviors. They can be dissociative, with amnesia for traumatic events. And they can feel ineffective, damaged for life, overresponsible for their problems, and consequently full of shame. Relationally, they may find it hard to trust anyone, hard to believe that anyone can understand them, and be prone to revictimization (if you can't trust anyone, you don't know what trustworthy looks like). They can be untrustworthy themselves, from being unable to keep commitments to being outright violent. Many have somatic symptoms: stomachaches, chronic pain, asthma or heart palpitations, dissociative conversion symptoms (e.g., numb body parts or hysterical blindness), or pain in their reproductive organs. They may feel that either they are hopeless or the world is. They may have little tolerance for or ability to feel happiness. The following is a vignette of development from DTD to DESNOS.

Developmental Trauma Disorder

You were bad. If you weren't, your mom would have looked you in the eyes. She'd have picked you up when you cried, and played the peek-a-boo game with you. At first, when she didn't respond, you'd try hard to get her attention, first being your cutest, then screaming. Nothing worked. You went dorsal, spacing out. It turned out that spacing out was a useful trick. When your dad starting doing sex on you, first you'd get mobilized: scared, waiting, waiting, waiting for the pain. Then you'd space out again. It worked pretty well. It even worked for the beatings, after they got going. After he was done, you felt like a dishrag, unable to move. During their fights, you'd start out tense, fearful, then sink back into that daze, if they didn't focus on you.

As you grew up, you learned to cope. You went to school, played, studied. You were like a different person when you were out of the house. But sometimes the inside life intruded on your outside life. You couldn't have close friends because everyone seemed scary. You couldn't say no to anyone about anything, because you couldn't say no at home. And anyway, you were supposed to rely on yourself, nobody else. Once in a while, all the rage would come out on somebody, usually someone you cared about. They'd do something little and you'd blow, saying terrible things. For a while, they would look to you like they were totally evil. Later, they wouldn't seem so awful to you, and you'd feel totally ashamed about how you were to them.

Sometimes you felt numb. Sometimes the smallest things could bring up huge anger or fear, for no good reason. Sometimes it felt like there was a huge hole in your stomach that could never get filled. It helped to eat and eat and eat. Sometimes, when the feelings were too big or the numbness too pervasive, you'd yank on your hair, or smash your fist on your leg. It was strange that hurting made you feel better. If it was really bad, sometimes you used a knife.

The headaches started when you were little. They were constant. Sometimes your ears would buzz, too. And most of the time, if you paid attention to it, your stomach hurt. It made it hard to study or even pay attention. Feeling too much or not feeling anything were like screens between you and the world.

There was nothing to do about it. The abuse is what you were for. You were there to not get in Mom's way, and to help Dad by taking all his rage and sex. And you always failed. Mom was still depressed. Dad was still angry. You failed at the only things you were there to do. If you had been a good person, it would have been different. But you were born a failure.

People say now, "Why didn't you do anything?" Like go to the cops. Why? What's the use? The parents would deny everything. Nothing would happen. And who would believe you? Even if they did, who else would have wanted you?

Disorders of Extreme Stress Not Otherwise Specified

You grew up and got madder. Mad at other people, mad at yourself. Sometimes you're mad enough or hopeless enough to try to kill yourself, and that's become one more thing that you've tried and failed. Since you got away from the parents, you cry more. When you do cry, it's really scary and out of control. Sometimes when the feelings start, it's like you're not you. You're just watching yourself cry from somewhere else. It's like when you used to float up to the ceiling when he was having sex on you.

You've connected with some other people, the wrong people, of course. There must be a sign on your back, "Only dates assholes." It's so intense and wonderful in the beginning, before it goes bad. And when it goes bad, you still need them. When they're not beating you up, you can hurt yourself. You know how to cut just deep enough for maximum effect. You've got scars upon scars upon scars. It might be the only thing you're good at. When you get your tattoos, it's like getting someone else to do it for you.

You don't think much about when you were at home. In fact, if people ask, you can barely remember what it was like. If you try to talk about it, the words don't come out very well. The therapist says, "Incoherent narrative." Whatever that means. Sometimes, you'll totally switch. You'll get so mad, or so scared, for no good reason, that it doesn't feel like you. And there's no way to put on the brakes. You just leave, either by spacing out or by yelling and walking out. Failing again.

Even though you're trying the therapy thing, you know it won't work. Nothing will. You're such a loser that you haven't been able to keep a job, a relationship, or even a friendship. Who would want you? And nobody understands you. Who could? And what's the point, really? You can't even do simple things that the therapist asks for. "Stay with that feeling." "Tell me what it is." "Tell me what happened." Nothing. A loser.

The headaches and the ear buzzing have gotten worse, especially when you try to think about the past. It hurts "down there" a lot of the time. And speaking of "down there," whenever you try to "do it," you end up thinking it's your father. That's just sick.

It won't get better. And you're running out of options. Life sucks. It's hopeless. You're hopeless.

CLINICAL WRAP-UP

All of these disorders are treatable and curable. This book shows you the modalities that therapists use to work with the range of traumatized clients, from simple one-event PTSD to the chronic accumulation of minor traumas and poor attachment, to the most complex dissociative disorders. As a trauma therapist you'll get to enjoy watching your well-attached clients with few other traumas clear their one-event trauma in a matter of weeks, no longer plagued by nightmares, flashbacks, and a feeling of helplessness. You'll feel the satisfaction of watching your more complex clients learn to stay in the room as they tolerate their affect, see themselves and others in a realistic light, set limits, live in the now, and connect to others from their authentic, whole selves. You'll get to experience the deep satisfactions inherent in digging deeply into your therapeutic toolbox and digging in for the long run with complex dissociative clients while they stabilize, learn to tolerate all of their memories and their connection with you and all of themselves, clear the trauma, integrate the parts, and grow into a new life.

TRAUMA RESOURCES

Judith Herman, *Trauma and Recovery* (Basic Books, 1992). A groundbreaking book about the effects of violence and how to treat them.

Glenn Shiraldi, *The Post-Traumatic Stress Disorder Sourcebook* (Lowell House, 2000). A user-friendly book for nonprofessionals with good tips for professionals.

Bessel van der Kolk, Alexander McFarlane, and Lars Weisaeth edited a field-changing book about the effects and treatment of trauma: *Traumatic Stress: The Effects of Overwhelming Experience on the Mind, Body and Society* (Guilford, 1966).

Marion Solomon and Daniel Siegel's *Healing Trauma* (Norton, 2006) has almost everything, presented by some of the best researchers and therapists in the field. The chapters are densely packed with information and give you strong descriptions of the neurology, affect, and many kinds of therapy for trauma with an emphasis on attachment issues and the therapeutic relationship.

CHAPTER TWO

Dissociation

When you banged your elbow, it exploded with pain. At first, your brain turned on the adrenaline and you swore or jumped around. Soon, your endogenous (internally created) opioids began pouring into your brain. As the opioids hit pain receptors, the pain began to ebb away and calmed down. You stopped swearing and jumping. You decided whether or not to put ice on your elbow and went on with your day. If your elbows were constantly getting whacked, a reflex would develop and your brain would helpfully start pouring on the opioids as you approached the elbow-banging situation.

Even before we're born, experience builds neural connections in our brains. As we continue to grow, experience, and learn, these conglomerations of neurons strengthen into pathways. We have preprogrammed pathways for eating, connecting with others, avoiding or confronting danger, and dealing with pain. When a trauma is big enough or happens often enough, we may develop strong, reflexive pathways of response that act separately from our most conscious, thinking, planning brain. Trauma-based reflexively triggered neural networks of emotional (Panksepp, 1998) or action-oriented (van der Hart, Nijenhuis, & Steele, 2006) neural systems are the basis of dissociative responses.

According to Bennett Braun (1988), dissociation can be seen as a continuum. "Normal" dissociation includes the ability to experience hypnotic states, including the "driving 10 miles without remembering anything about it" state and spacing out when we're bored. Most people have dissociative states or "parts" that are well-trodden neural networks pertaining to an age, situation, or activity. In Braun's and my opinion, PTSD is a dissociative disorder in which the dissociated affect, images, body sensations, and cognitions from the traumatic event intrude upon present consciousness. The further along the continuum, the more dissociation. Further along the continuum, past PTSD, Braun has the *Diagnostic and Statistical Manual (DSM)* official dissociative disorders, including dissociative disorder not otherwise specified (DDNOS), amnesic fugue states, and dissociative identity disorder (DID), formerly known as multiple personality disorder.

Avoidance or Dissociation?

Nearly every trauma theory and therapy addresses avoidance. Most describe the phenomenon of trauma survivors who avoid thinking about distressing events and anything that could trigger memories or flashbacks of distressing events. Most contain mechanisms that directly confront avoidance. The cognitive therapies target the thoughts about avoidance: "I can't stand the memories." "I'll go crazy if I think about it." Exposure and experiential therapies direct clients to reexperience aspects of the trauma, the narrative, the sensations, the emotions, the cognitions, or all aspects.

Avoidance is not always dissociative. Some avoidance is conscious and choiceful. "Since the accident, it gives me the willies to go by that corner. Let's go another way." Or, "I don't want to talk about it!" When avoidance is reflexive, it may be a dissociative phenomenon, the conditioned response of endogenous opiates rewarding the brain for avoiding the distress (Goleman, 1985; Lanius, 2005). In dissociation, you will see clients droop into semiconscious states, become incoherent, become flooded with flashbacks or internal voices, forget what they're talking about, or completely switch to another part of themselves in a reflexive, unconscious reaction to a question.

The Structural Dissociation Theory

Onno van der Hart, Ellert Nijenhuis, and Kathy Steele (2006) have developed a versatile model for understanding and treating the effects of trauma. Their structural dissociation theory covers everything from simple PTSD to DESNOS and some personality disorders common in traumatized individuals, to the most polyfragmented DID client.

Primary Dissociation

The ideal, well-attached, untraumatized person is able to regulate and tolerate affect (feelings), behaves appropriately in daily life, connects well with others, isn't avoidant of experiences inside the body or safe experiences outside the body, and feels more or less like the same person across experiences. This ideal person is less susceptible to simple PTSD or any other level of dissociation than people with poor attachment, poor self-regulation, and prior stress and trauma. During a traumatic enough event even an ideally healthy person will experience an integrative failure in the face of overwhelming stress that manifests in a division between an emotional part (EP) of the personality that holds the affect, cognition, somatic sensations, and the rest of the experience of the trauma, and an apparently normal part (ANP) of the personality that avoids the trauma (van der Hart et al., 2006). EPs "contain the memories of experiences that are originally overwhelming, remain dysfunctionally stored neurologically, and continue to press for activation in conscious experience as relivings" (Bergmann, 2008, p. 64). Bergmann writes about Panksepp's "emotional operating systems, as defined by genetically coded neural circuits in animal and human brains that generate well-organized behavior sequences," which can be evoked by the sight of food, a loved one, a rival or a predator, or even by electrical stimulation of specific areas of the brain:

1. The seeking system, which mediates interest in and exploration of the environment, food seeking, warmth, and sexual gratification (an ANP correlate)

2. The fear system, which mediates hypervigilance, flight, freeze, or collapse (EP)

3. The rage system, which mediates fight (EP)

4. The panic system, which mediates attachment cry, which precedes clinging (EP) (p. 64)

EPs are based in defense-related "action-systems" that "involve an innate readiness or tendency to act" that have been hindered "from a natural progression toward integration" (Steele, van der Hart, & Nijenhuis, 2005, p. 20) and become chronic, reflexive, inappropriate responses to present life circumstances.

The Apparently Normal Part is guided by action systems that handle any activities that let life go on: working, cooking, parenting, playing, and connecting with other people. For the ANP, the EPs feel like an outside intrusion on the self. The ANP tends to avoid external cues (scene of the accident, driving, etc.) and internal cues (thinking about the accident, feeling too much, or anything that triggers an EP state). I like the way that the structural dissociation model explains this phenomenon as phobias of traumatic memories that keep EP material or triggering from intruding on the ANP. Every successful trauma therapy overtly deals with getting clients who are affect avoidant or phobic to approach, own, and experience traumatic material.

PRETRAUMATIZED PERSON
fragments during simple trauma into:
Emotional Part of the Personality and Apparently Normal Part

Primary Structural Dissociation: one ANP and one EP (PTSD)

Secondary Structural Dissociation: one ANP and more than one EP
(DESNOS, DDNOS, some borderline personality disorder)

Tertiary: More than one ANP and more than one EP (DID)

Two months after returning from Iraq, John feels okay some of the time. He can do his job and enjoy some aspects of his life. But he still has nightmares. And when he sees a car coming through the intersection or people standing around on the street, he gets agitated and hypervigilant. He avoids talking about and even tries to avoid thinking about the dangerous situations he faced in the Middle east, but the images and thoughts are constantly intruding, affecting his functioning.

Secondary Dissociation: One ANP and Two or More EPs

Children with Developmental Trauma Disorder (DTD) or adults with Complex Traumatic Stress Disorders/Disorders of Extreme Stress or Dissociative Disorders Not Otherwise Specified (DDNOS) develop another layer of dissociation. Each EP tendency involves an action system, like seeking, panic, or rage, that shapes what the EP attends to and how it behaves and feels, and that when repeatedly reinforced with new trauma builds a wide neural pathway to a strong defensive traumatic reaction. The EPs are fixated (or stuck) in the defensive mobilized and immobilized states that occurred during the time of the trauma. The mobilized intrusive states can include hypervigilance, freeze, flight, fight, cling, and panic. The immobilized EP states include numbness, anesthesia/surrender/submit, shut down, and a recuperative swoon state. DESNOS clients can have sensitive triggers, flying into a rage or huddling on the floor when a seemingly slight provocation cues a strong EP state, (e.g., fight or collapse).

EPs can also engage in daily life activities, but in a trauma-related way, such as the "slut" part that has sex or the anorexic part that refuses to eat because she feels sick to her stomach because of abuse memories, and so on. Generally in simple PTSD, an EP has physical defenses. In some secondary and tertiary dissociation, some EPs may have additional daily life functions that have become subsumed as traumatic reactions. And some EPs are fantasy based so that the defense that was not able to be enacted during the trauma is the major one, for instance, a part that believes he killed his father in rage, or that wants to kill him in the present, when in fact, the child was unable to safely express anger at all during the time of the trauma.

In DDNOS and DID, some dissociative parts, guided or mediated by action systems, become elaborate and relatively autonomous, with ages, job descriptions, and sometimes names. And autonomy can either be external (switching) or internal (passive influence). Lots of parts are elaborated internally but do not fully switch externally.

I make sense of most attachment, personality, *DSM* Axis II disorders as combinations of EP physical defense states and ANP defenses against particular affects and states. I see narcissistic personality disorder as a combination of a shame-avoiding ANP with a fight EP that may alternate with a shut down or depressed EP on the side. People with borderline personality disorder (BPD) may have a combination of a fight, a panic, a cling, and an immobilized submit EP with an ANP of varying strength. In the same vein, dependent personality = panic + cling. Paranoid = mobilized flight + fight. Schizoid = flight + immobilized shut down states. Of course, personality disorders are more complex than these simple equations, but an awareness of the structural dissociation model can aid in the diagnosis and functional understanding of a complex client.

DESNOS Client with BPD

Julie had a rotten childhood. She was the youngest child of two narcissistic, alcoholic parents, and had older siblings who either ignored her or, in the case of her two older brothers, sexually abused her. Her father was yeller and a beater. Her mother was critical and dismissive. Her family moved a lot and thus constantly broke her attachments to people and places.

As a result of her poor attachment, subsequent poor emotional self-regulation, and a frightening childhood, Julie developed several reflexive EP states. At 33 she connected with me, her therapist, quickly—too quickly. Her mobilized EP cling state was my first tip-off to her diagnosis. If she felt threatened, her fight state instantaneously appeared and I became "bad." And if faced with a potential loss, or an angry boyfriend, she collapsed into an immobilized, dorsal vagal, depressive state. Julie's ANP presentation was delightful. She was well-groomed, funny, engaging, and cooperative. She was skilled in her computer systems work, but often lost jobs because her fight state emerged whenever she was challenged by authority. Her relationships were stormy. Her cling EP found boyfriends with qualities of her parents: narcissism, substance abuse, and rage. Her volatile boyfriends would kindle state shifts in Julie, until the relationships exploded, then ended, and she would sink into a deep dorsal depressed EP state for months. She came into my office during one of these states.

Tertiary Dissociation: DID With Two or More ANPs and Two or More EPs

In extreme dissociation, DID, the neural pathways become multi-lane highways. As in DDNOS, dissociative parts that are guided or mediated by action systems become elaborate and relatively autonomous. But there is also more than one ANP, each with separate daily life functions. I knew a DID person in whom one ANP part manifested in math class, and another in history class. As an adult, she had ANP parts that did different pieces of her complicated work. This is a good example of dissociation being used to cope with daily life rather than with the trauma.

Mobilized EPs might be "the ones that run away," fighters, and holders of different vehement affects including rage and panic. Some may have names and know their origins. Others are fragments, less elaborated and autonomous. For survivors of intense abuse, there may be mobilized parts for anticipating the abuse and experiencing the beginning of it; immobilized parts that "went dorsal" while being raped or beaten; separate parts that hold the anger, the hopelessness, the shame, and the fear; a "part that got away" and went to a fantasy place during the abuse; an immobilized part that lies around in a nearly unconscious, postabuse state, and an ANP-related part that cleaned up afterward and made sure that no one knew. Some parts may not know that other parts exist. Others may understand themselves to be part of a system.

DID Client

Bonnie's mother had been sexually abused by a family member and was unable to attach to and contain her energetic child. When Bonnie's father died, the 3-year-old went to a foster home in which the children were systematically and ritually abused. During the abuse, Bonnie split into several EPs: Sad Baby, who lived in the submit state, held the physical memory and sensations of the abuse, and felt hopeless; B.T., who held the feistiness and anger and who went off to "Mother Goose Land" during the abuse; parts that identified with the power of the abusers; and several other parts. Years after the ritual abuse, 8-year-old Bonnie was abused by her grandfather and developed more splits. When I met her, in her late 30s, her ANPs alternated between a bright 12-year-old part, a feisty teenage part, and a serious adult. She instantly switched to raging, seductive, or submissive EPs with the slightest provocation.

CLINICAL WRAP-UP

There are many ways to think about trauma and dissociation. The polyvagal theory addresses part of the effect of the trauma on the body and the brain. Other trauma researchers and theorists talk more about the hippocampus, the amygdala, the secretion of stress hormones, and the interaction between the dozens of systems that mediate trauma, dissociation, and healing. In the section on treatment for complex trauma cases, structural dissociation has its own chapter. If you want to know about the assessment of dissociation, read Chapter 3, "Assessment." If you want to know more about the neurobiology of trauma and dissociation, structural dissociation, and ego state therapies, read the following books.

Uri Bergmann's chapter, "She's Come Undone: A Neurological Exploration of Dissociative Disorders" in Forgash and Copeley's book *Healing the Heart of Trauma and Dissociation with EMDR Ego State Therapy* (Springer, 2008). The most succinct and clear explanation that I've seen of the biology of dissociation.

J. Panksepp, *Affective Neuroscience: The Foundations of Human and Animal Emotions* (Oxford University Press, 1998).

A. N. Schore, *Affect Regulation and the Origin of the Self: The Neurobiology of Emotional Development* (Erlbaum, 1994).

D. J. Siegel, *The Developing Mind: Toward a Neurobiology of Interpersonal Experience* (Guilford, 1999).

DISSOCIATION RESOURCES

Van der Hart, Nijenhuis, and Steele, *The Haunted Self: Structural Dissociation and the Treatment of Chronic Traumatization* (Norton, 2006). It's dense, the language is sometimes difficult, and it covers phenomena that I haven't seen anywhere else. The writers explain Pierre Janet's still vital theory of dissociation and stages of treatment. If you work with dissociation, you must read this book.

Colin Ross, *Dissociative Identity Disorder: Diagnosis, Clinical Features, and Treatment of Multiple Personality* (Wiley & Sons, 1997). A classic.

James A. Chu, *Rebuilding Shattered Lives: The Responsible Treatment of Complex Post-Traumatic and Dissociative Disorders* (Wiley, 1998). Another classic.

Courtois and Ford (eds.), *Treating Complex Post-Traumatic Stress Disorders.* (Guilford, 2009). It covers all the bases. An important book.

The International Society for the Study of Trauma and Dissociation's Web site (http://www.isst-d.org/) is an information clearinghouse, membership organization, and list serve for all topics pertaining to trauma, trauma therapy, and dissociation. The ISSTD throws a great yearly conference, packed with information on assessing, understanding, and treating trauma and dissociation.

Part II

GETTING READY

CHAPTER THREE

Assessment

In early sessions, we therapists need to find out, first, who our clients are, and second, how traumas have impacted their lives. Traumatic events affect people differently. We are genetically endowed with idiosyncratic systems of affect and arousal modulation. These systems are impacted by the nurturing we receive and our individual experiences. When we plan our assessment, we need to take all of that into account.

I organize my assessments around Maureen Kitchur's (2005) strategic developmental model (SDM). Before delving into Kitchur or talking about obvious trauma, I'll describe some other components of assessment.

TEMPERAMENT

We are born with distinct temperaments. We are predisposed to be night owls or early risers, introverts or extroverts, stolidly calm or reactively nervous. People can be born with predispositions for depression, anxiety, or bipolar disorder. These conditions and our less pathological temperaments predict some of our perceptions and responses to trauma.

Working with couples, I've heard at least 50 versions of the following story. Here's one I have permission to tell.

While the tour bus lurched back and forth across the Costa Rican highway, Renee gave up reading her book and started to enjoy the wild ride down the long hill. David, at her side, clutched the armrest, pulled his shoulders up around his ears, and swore that he'd never, ever, take a Central American bus again. When they hit the big bump, Renee whooped and David screamed. Back home, Renee barely remembers the careening bus. When she does, it's as a funny story. David still has a trauma reaction. His body was in a hyperaroused sympathetic (and depressed ventral vagal) state during the ride. His amygdala and hippocampus were lit up. His brain told him that he was going to die. It took him days to calm down after the ride. When anything reminds David of the bus ride, he has a full PTSD reexperiencing of the event. When asked about it 9 years later, he looks distressed and says, "Oh no! Don't make me think of that!"

Slim, energetic David is from a constitutionally anxious family. Two of his siblings have full-blown obsessive-compulsive disorder. The other, a workaholic, uses alcohol to medicate his anxiety. David fits Elaine Aron's (1996) definition of a highly sensitive person (HSP): easily overwhelmed by stimulus, creative, and needing quiet time alone every day to recuperate from social and environmental stimuli. He's friendly and social, capable of deep intimacy with Renee and his friends, but still introverted. He is the "designated worrier" in his marriage, leaving less to chance than his more placid partner. Renee is descended from rowdy, big-bodied people, is not phased by most external stimuli, and is most definitely extroverted. On their travels, she talks to strangers, while he wanders, alone, taking pictures of the landscape. Their wild bus ride shows the differential effects of the same stimuli on two very different people.

Some people are born to be anxious. Endogenous anxiety disorders create their own trauma. Panic disorder is the worst. With or without external triggers, people with panicked bodies react as if they were in the worst kind of danger and then continue to shake, sweat, and hyperventilate, despite cognitive awareness of safety. Most panic sufferers feel as if they are totally out of control, or even dying. Some would rather die than experience another attack. They have PTSD responses to their own visceral experiences and any perceived triggers. When we treat clients with panic disorder, we often need to target the external triggers (if any), internal triggers, and the frightening panic response itself, before going on to external traumas.

All sufferers of endogenous or genetically based anxiety disorders suffer from high arousal; they are likely to have a greater depression of ventral vagal responses and a greater expression of sympathetic responses to distressing stimuli. They feel more distress at the time of the event and cannot calm down as fast as other people. When clients come in clearly traumatized by small stimuli, and there is no past trauma that's being currently triggered, suspect an anxiety disorder.

Some bipolar and depression sufferers have heightened or out-of-control anxiety. Small distresses may turn into subjectively major trauma for these folks. First-degree relatives (kids and siblings) of bipolar sufferers often display anxiety disorders. Keep your eyes open during your intake.

Some people are born to be slow. From birth, they don't show much affect and have tendencies toward depression or dysthymia and the shut down, immobilized, dorsal vagal kind of dissociation. These folks may hold their trauma symptoms deep inside. When traumatized, they just look (and feel) more depressed. They feel still. They inhabit the dorsal vagal, immobilized end of the scale. They are sometimes characterized as difficult clients because they don't give the social engagement that many therapists crave. They rarely volunteer much about their inner life and need a lot of questions to express themselves. You need to ask explicit and specific questions and be patient with the answers when working with depressed or depressive people. And you need to find ways of finding what combination of nature, nurture, and trauma created the depression in your still, heavy-feeling client.

Genetics are only one cause for depression. Find out if your depressed client is drinking, on benzodiazapines, has a low thyroid, or is going through menopause. Find out if your anxious client is drinking five double lattes or is hopped up on sugar, has an overactive thyroid or is taking Adderall or other speed-like medications (Shapiro, 2009b). And keep in mind that trauma can impact people no matter what their temperament, biology, or substance intake.

TEMPERAMENT ASSESSMENT

Observation

- How does this client seem? Nervous? Calm? Depressed? Spaced out?
- Is he a skinny, nervous person? (generalized anxiety disorder or HSP)

- Is she hypervigilant about your response to her? (social anxiety)
- Is he sitting like a lump? (depression, illness, exhaustion, dissociation)
- Does she avoid different subjects, going on at length about the minutiae of unrelated things? (obsessive-compulsive, obsessive-compulsive personality, or attention deficit disorder, or just plain avoidance)
- Does he change the subject every few seconds? (mania or attention deficit disorder)
- Are there any other signs of major depression, mania, or anxiety disorders?

Questions for the Client

- You seem a little anxious. Is that normal for you, since the car accident, or because of this therapy situation?
- How far back can you remember being anxious?
- Have you ever had a panic attack? When did they start? What are they like?
- Have you ever taken medications for anxiety? What kind?
- Are you still on them? How are they working?
- Is there anyone else in your family who has anxiety? What are they like?
- Any depression, bipolar, or manic depression in your family? Any schizophrenia?
- Was anyone hospitalized for emotional issues? On medications? Do you know what kind?
- Have you had any of these diagnoses?
- If pertinent: How long have you been anxious, depressed, or feeling angry? Did the feelings start after the traumatic event, or have you felt that way for a long time? Do they come and go, or hang around all the time?

CULTURE

Everyone is born into a cultural context. We all have a race, an ethnicity, a social class, a gender, and a sexual orientation. Some of us fit into our expected niches. Many of us don't.

Know who you're dealing with. And watch out for your own projections about who your clients are. Acknowledge (to yourself) your biases and prejudices about the person with whom you're working. Then work to know more about your particular client. Be aware of the chronic trauma that dysfunctional sex role expectations, directed hatred, institutionalized discrimination, and social expectations can have on individuals who don't fit the dominant picture of who to be.

While you're doing your other assessments, keep these things in mind:

- What kind of cultural and familial expectations does your client hold? What is the dominant feeling? Pride? Shame? Fear of being hurt? Rejected? Beaten up? Shunned? Never measuring up? Loved only for fitting in, without truly being seen?
- Social class: Did the family fit into their milieu? Did your client fit in? What were the class-based expectations? "We must always look perfect"? "We'll never amount to anything"?
- Race: Were there chronic stressors tied to race? Specific discrete traumas? What were the family's expectations? The neighborhood's? The culture's?
- Migration: Where did your client come from? Was the move traumatic? Was the client fleeing discrimination, economic hardship, or genocide in her original culture? Is there a disconnect between social expectations in the homeland and this culture? Does your client feel like a full part of this society? How long did that take?
- Sexual orientation: Is she "out"? Scared to tell the family? Are there constant fears of being discovered or being discounted? Discrete traumatic incidents? Bashing? Did he have a supportive family and a happy gay relationship that has nothing to do with the trauma that brought him to therapy?
- Gender: Does he fit the stereotype of a "real man"? Does she fit the expectation of a female in her culture? What did it cost them try to fit in or to be so different? Were there lowered expectations because she was a girl? What kinds of discrimination has she run into?
- Religion: What did his religion tell your client about himself?

Did it bring trauma? Solace and support? Discrimination? An impossible standard to live by? A strong identification with a community? A strong sense of values?

- Appearance: Does she hate herself for her body type? Has he been humiliated for being too slight to play football?
- Disability: How did other people treat this difference? How did it make your client feel separate?
- Family: What were the family messages about self, about the larger society, and about being enough? Do "Smiths never give up"? Do they always fail? Does the client feel safe in and a full part of the family? Is the client estranged or seen as the different one or the caretaker to the family?
- What of all of the above brings up your own issues with a client? What projections do you need to keep in check, in order to truly see the client in front of you? What kind of research do you need to do about this client's culture or situation? And how do you keep yourself from blindly laying what you learn on a client whom it may not fit?

Laura Brown's *Cultural Competence in Trauma Therapy: Beyond the Flashback* (APA, 2008), covers all these bases.

ATTACHMENT AND AFFECT REGULATION

Our brains are predisposed to learn how to regulate our emotions. Our interactions with caregivers allow that learning to take place (Schore, 1994; Siegel, 1999). When our parent or caregiver mirrors our affect, soothes us, or appropriately responds to us, we learn that we can expect a response, that we are worth responding to, and that we can be soothed. In the meantime, we build the neural hardware for handling our emotions. If we have a depressed, addicted, overwhelmed, or angry caregiver, we might learn that help is unreliable or unavailable, that we aren't worth it anyway, and that our brains don't have good ways to calm us down. Without the brain hardware for calming down, some of us learn to reflexively dissociate when emotions, even good emotions, arise. We come to be at the mercy of every emotion that runs through us, either dissociating or overreacting to strong affect, whether it is positive or negative. (Think about histrionic or borderline personality disorders.) If those emotions run through us over and over, they build the hardware for strong state-specific reactions and poor or nonexistent self-regulation.

People with poor affect regulation react strongly to distress and may have stronger and more pernicious PTSD symptoms from newer trauma. Poor attachment experiences often accompany early abuse and physical neglect—the Triple Crown of devastating psychological consequences. Watch for bone-deep trauma reactions (including dissociation) in people with disordered attachment.

ATTACHMENT ASSESSMENT

Observation

- Can this client connect? Make eye contact?
- Does she respond appropriately to me? To humor? To serious inquiry?
- Is his narrative coherent, when he's talking about childhood? How is it not holding together? (Mary Main [1991] found that coherency of narrative in discussing childhood was the strongest indication of attachment style and level of dissociation.)
- How do I feel in the presence of this person? Comfortable? Defensive? Distant? Connected? (This is often a reflection of what's going on in the client.)
- As she talks about her life, does she seem like her actual age, or younger? Does it feel like she's switching from one neural network (age or part) to another?

Questions for the Client

- What was your family going through when you were a kid? Any deaths, losses, divorces, moves, big changes? What was the effect of these changes on your parents? On you?
- Who took care of you? One parent? Both? Paid caregivers? Relatives? What was that like?
- How did your family deal with feelings?
- What happened when you cried? Got mad? Needed something? Ran around making noise?
- Was there anyone who made you feel treasured or adored?

- Was there anyone who made you feel like you weren't wanted? That you shouldn't have been born? That you were too much to deal with?

AFFECT TOLERANCE

People who can tolerate strong feelings are the best candidates for any trauma therapy. Clients who reflexively dissociate or actively avoid affect may need specific preparation before tackling their traumas. Both temperament and attachment experience impact affect regulation. After intense trauma, PTSD can dysregulate the emotions of the calmest, most well-raised person. During assessment, you want to know if the dysregulated emotions and affect phobias (van der Hart et al., 2006) are specific to recent trauma or chronic manifestations of temperament or attachment issues. You want to know if clients can more or less comfortably feel sad, mad, glad, scared, and proud. If they can't tolerate their affect, you need to develop a working hypothesis about why they can't. Is it nature, nurture, or the current trauma?

The Window of Tolerance

Traumatized people are vulnerable to hyperaroused or mobilized states with increased sensation, emotional reactivity, hypervigilance, intrusive imagery, and disorganized cognitive processing and hypoaroused or immobilized states with numbing of sensations and emotion, disabled cognitive processing, and reduced physical movement (Ogden et al., 2006). Between these autonomic zones lies the window of tolerance (Ogden et al., 2006), the optimal arousal zone from which people experience "various intensities of emotional and physiological arousal without disrupting the functioning of the system" (Siegel, 1999, p. 253). Therapists must assist clients to stay in the window of tolerance so that they can think, feel, and process through their traumas, without being either overwhelmed or shut down. Early in therapy, we need to assess clients' range and tolerance of affect and autonomic states. Throughout the therapy, we need to collaborate with clients to keep them in their window of tolerance: able to think, feel, and process their emotions.

AFFECT TOLERANCE ASSESSMENT

Observation

- Is his affect appropriate to the material?
- Does she space out or freak out when a feeling begins to arise?
- Is he embarrassed by showing feeling? (Is this a gender issue: "Boys don't cry," or family training to "buck up," or something else?)
- Can she tolerate her positive affect? Smile? Laugh appropriately? Feel pride?
- What is his window of tolerance for affect? What amount of affect or arousal causes him to shut down, or get too distressed?

Questions for the Client

- What's it like to cry now? Do you cry? Does it feel manageable, like you can stop if you want? Do you feel ashamed to cry? (Watch for gender differences here.)
- How have your feelings changed since the event? (If there was a recent trauma.)
- What were your feelings like before the event?
- When you think of what happened or get triggered, do you ever feel shut down? (Check for depression, too.)
- When you think of what happened or get triggered, do you ever feel so agitated you can't stand it?
- Describe a time when you felt proud of yourself. What do you feel in your body when you think of that? (If they can't think of a proud time, consider attachment problems. If they can think of a time but can't feel it now, it could be PTSD-related or other depression.)
- What happens when you get mad? Can you express it? Do you feel in control of yourself when you're angry? Does it feel safe to be angry?
- Have you ever experienced a big loss? Tell me about it. (Watch for appropriate or inappropriate affect.)

DISSOCIATION ASSESSMENT

It's easy to diagnose DID when your client of several sessions changes stance and voice and asks, "Who are you? Where is this? What are we doing here?" (showing huge state changes and obvious amnesia between states). Most signs of dissociation are more subtle. The more you know about dissociation, the more you automatically watch for its markers. You'll notice when your new client:

1. Spaces out easily
2. Loses coherency when speaking about childhood events (Main, 1991; Siegel, 1999, 2007)
3. Can't remember much of childhood years
4. Begins to use different voices, inflections, or age-specific language
5. Abruptly switches from calm discussion to a hostile, terrified, shut down, or disorganized state
6. Is easily triggered into feelings of abandonment, defensiveness, or clinginess
7. Subtly or not so subtly changes stance and expression in a "weird" way
8. Has otherwise unexplained headaches or pelvic pain
9. Doesn't connect with you
10. Shows inappropriate affect when discussing distressing events
11. Speaks in the third person about the self
12. Forgets appointments, despite a good therapeutic relationship

Since few clients announce that they have secondary dissociation (personality, character, or Axis II disorders) or DID or DDNOS (tertiary dissociation), some clinicians use diagnostic tools to screen every client for dissociative disorders. Others use these tools only when they can't come to a diagnosis without them.

Here are some helpful screening tools:

1. The Dissociative Experiences Scale (DES) is a 28-item questionnaire on which the client reports on the prevalence of common and not-so-common dissociative experiences. It's easily rated for

degrees of dissociation from PTSD to DID (Bernstein & Putnam, 1986).

2. The Dissociative Disorders Interview Schedule (DDIS) is a comprehensive 132-item highly structured interview. It evaluates depression, borderline personality disorder, and all levels of dissociation. Download it (for free) at www.rossinst.com/dddquest .htm from Dr. Colin Ross (1997), its creator. Just by reading it, you will become a better diagnostician.

3. Somatoform Questionnaire (SDQ): Available in 20-item and 5-item versions, the SDQ evaluates somatoform dissociation (physical and sensory experiences) and other dissociative disorders. Available from Ellert Nijenhuis's Web site: www.enijenhuis.nl/index.html

MAUREEN KITCHUR'S STRATEGIC DEVELOPMENTAL MODEL

If your client has an easy temperament, great early attachment, good affect regulation, no early trauma, and only a few recent traumas, you're good to go with almost any decent trauma therapy. Since only 5% of my traumatized clients fit that category, I use Maureen Kitchur's (2005) SDM model to assess the rest. Kitchur developed this model for EMDR practitioners, but, with some tweaking, the SDM can work as the basis for any kind of trauma assessment. The main function of the model is "to interrupt the current problem by resolving the developmental conditions that have been perpetuating the symptoms" (p. 10).

Maureen Kitchur has given me permission to share her system with you.

SDM Assessment Components

1. "The SDM encourages deliberate utilization of transference to facilitate reparative attachment and encourages deep attunement between client and therapist." In other words, it creates the safety and good therapeutic attachment that is the basis for all trauma therapy.

2. "The SDM provides clinicians with a structured, directive

history-taking and assessment format that quickly yields a developmental hypothesis or template, from which it becomes possible to formulate a macro-therapy plan that addresses the experiences and developmental interruptions contributory to pathology or dysfunction in a client's life."

3. "The SDM provides highly sensitive, facilitative, flexible language that assures clients of their safety and rapidly engages both the client's conscious and unconscious resources and cooperation . . . allowing the client to align with the therapist's confident vision of healing" (Kitchur, 2005, pp. 11–12).

So, while you're doing the assessment, you're not just getting the facts, you're opening up to understand the person.

> By being consistent and trustworthy, keeping commitments, being punctual, being unconditionally accepting, and maintaining boundaries, while at the same time being warm, caring, and available, we teach trust and model good ego boundaries. When we are "real" with clients, model a range of affects, and facilitate and sometimes induce affect, we have a fertile environment in which to teach affect recognition and promote affect development. When we model our comfort with intense affect, coach clients to express and articulate emotion, and teach self-soothing strategies . . . we facilitate the affect-regulation that truly is as Allan Schore (1994) terms it, "the foundation for the origin of the self." (p. 14)

How does Kitchur promote therapeutic attachment? She sits close, makes warm, expressive eye contact, and pays attention to the interplay of her client's and her own body language and to the qualities of her client's voice and her own. She has read Schore (1994, 2009) and Siegel (1999, 2003, 2007, 2009), as should you. She lets her clients know that they are going to tackle the trauma together.

How does she take a history? She draws a genogram, a family tree similar to McGoldrick and Gerson's (1985, 1999). While she draws, she asks "nosy, snoopy questions" to find out where the family comes from, who has been in it and is in it now, and how the dynamics have played out. Who is close to whom? Who doesn't speak to each other? She asks about class, ethnicity, moves, disruptions, and professions, with special attention to any event that has been "developmentally interruptive."

Kitchur asks open-ended questions throughout the genogram process:

- What was your grandfather/grandmother/and so on like?
- What was it like for your dad/mom/stepparent to grow up in his family?
- My favorite Kitchur questions are: So, with your dad/stepdad coming from that background, and mom/stepmom from hers, each of them fully formed people, what kind of marriage did they create and how did their individual "stuff" interact with each other's? How did their backgrounds shape the way they parented you and your siblings?
- What was it like to be the oldest/middle/youngest child?

Kitchur continues to ask questions until she, and the client, get a clear view of the family. Then she introduces the "nosy, snoopy questions": "Great, we've got a lot of the information and we'll need to map out a good treatment plan. I just have a few more nosy, snoopy questions that I ask everybody. These are questions about some of the tougher things you've lived through, or that you know have happened in your family, but fortunately I only need brief answers to these questions today—just a few words or sentences will tell me what we need to note on our genogram for future healing." She tells clinicians: "The therapist's style needs to be such that it models safety, nurturing, and, most importantly, self-regulation. Clients can experience that difficult material can be touched on, and the therapist's model of emotional equilibrium can be followed and even gradually internalized. Modeling and initiating this well-regulated survey of difficult material seeds an even more powerful unspoken message for the client: that they can handle the intense affect to come." Kitchur says to give appropriate comfort if big affect arises, but "generally, the pace set is one that allows the questions to be answered in a single setting."

Questions can include, and are not limited to, the following:

- Witness or victim of domestic violence, physical, sexual, emotional abuse, or military violence
- Alcohol, substance, or eating disorder problems in the family, self, or caregivers

- Neglect, abandonment, or separations (arrests, foster care, adoption, hospitalization)
- Separation, divorce, traumatic losses, scapegoating, serious accidents, or injuries
- Medical conditions or surgeries
- Pregnancy traumas (in grandmothers, mother, sisters if relevant, or self) including multiple births, abortions, miscarriages, SIDS, infertility, or birth defects
- Untimely moves or job losses; immigration
- Incarcerations, or victim or witness to crime
- Disasters (floods, fires, etc.)
- Peer or school traumas, or learning disabilities
- Religious trauma or abuse
- Workplace violence, harassment, stress, firings, layoffs, bad bosses

Abuse and violent relationships are depicted on the genogram by means of an arrow from the perpetrator to the victim. The type of abuse (physical, emotional or verbal, or sexual), the client's approximate age at the time of the trauma, and the general frequency of the abuse are noted along the arrow (Kitchur, 2005, pp. 20–21). (Because I think it's important to acknowledge the good stuff, in my color coding of the genogram, pink lines go between family members who adore each other, and I circle positive "developmentally impactful" events and resources with pink, too.) I circle all the alcoholics with one color, the depressives with another, and the PTSD sufferers with another. When clients can see the graphics of three or four generations of trauma, substance abuse, or mental illness in their families, it can be validating and shame busting. I'll often color code other issues, illnesses, professions, and identities. I'll plot everything from the prevalence of entrepreneurs or teachers to the presence of obesity, bipolar disorder, or ADD. This process makes these patterns manifest. Finally, Kitchur gathers contextual information including medical and therapy histories, substance history and current usage, medication history, supplements, and current nutrition.

In the one to three sessions that it takes to do an SDM intake, you get more than a clue about who your client is and the context of his or her historical and current life. You have an idea about the client's attachment style and ability to hold a coherent narrative (or not), including memories of past events. You have seen your client answer hard questions and have noticed how he or she tolerates and regulates the ensuing emotions. You can feel how the therapeutic relationship has grown, or not. And you begin to construct a theory of your client's therapy.

You can put a list of your client's goals and a list of the traumas that you will be tackling in different places on the page. Many of us list the traumas chronologically, the order in which we will clear them out.

Since particular therapies stress different areas of assessment, more detail is given in later chapters.

SDM Resources

Find Maureen Kitchur's strategic developmental model in Robin Shapiro (Ed.), *EMDR Solutions: Pathways to Healing* (pp. 8–56, Norton, 2005).

M. McGoldrick and R. Gerson, *Genograms in Family Assessment* (Norton, 1985).

M. McGoldrick and R. Gerson, *Genograms: Assessment and Intervention* (Norton, 1999).

Psychological Tests for PTSD and Dissociation

There are several assessment instruments for PTSD and dissociation. Here are two:

- PTSD Test, online at Healthy Place: http://www.healthyplace .com/psychological-tests/ptsd-test/
- The Penn Inventory for Posttraumatic Stress Disorder (Hammarburg, 1992)

Clinical Wrap-Up

For you beginning therapists who might be overwhelmed with the magnitude of assessment data, don't worry. It gets easier as you go along. You already assess people all day. The more you know about psychology, the deeper and more automatic your assessments become. Experienced therapists can often get a broad idea of their clients' strengths and deficits in the first few minutes. They pose themselves questions: "Just how dissociated is this guy?" or "Is this an inborn anxiety disorder or a trauma reaction or some of both?" and then look for the answers. The more knowledge and experience you have, the more you inform your intuition and the more you know what to look for, what to ask, and what to skip in the assessment process. It gets easier as you go along.

CHAPTER FOUR

Preparation

Assessment is one part of preparation for trauma work. Part of your assessment is knowing what your client wants to change. One way to find out is to ask, "When you lay me off for a job well done, what will be different?" Coach the client to be as specific as possible. Start at the first phone call: "When you come in, bring me your list of what you'd like to change." A typical list for a newly traumatized client will include comments such as: "I'll sleep better. No more nightmares. No flashbacks. I'll be less jumpy. I'll feel like myself again. I'll have my old self back. I'll be happy again." A list for a chronically traumatized client may be deeper: "I'll get along with people better. I'll like myself better. I'll feel like I belong. I won't automatically take care of everyone all the time. I won't be afraid all the time. I'll stop picking up jerks." Or, "I don't know what I want, but I know I'm a mess and I need to change."

Second, do your evaluation.

Third, after you have an understanding of who your client is and the depth of the trauma symptoms she or he experiences, you decide which therapy or combination of therapies will be most helpful. You may find, as you go along, that you switch modalities as you know your client better.

Fourth, you need to imagine a timeline for the therapy and talk with your client about the journey ahead. You need the client to understand and buy in to the plan. Use "we" language. Be as specific as you can about how you're thinking of the case. And give an outline about what the therapy might be.

A buy-in talk with the rare one-trauma client could go like this:

> Except for this car accident, you have had a low-trauma life. Your parents sound good. You've got a great family and good support. We need to get your brain and your body reprogrammed so that they know that the accident is over, you survived, and you're okay. It's going to take us some weeks to get there, but we'll use X technique, which I'll explain to you now.

A typical buy-in talk with a client who has a less-than-optimal but better-than-the-worst history might go like this:

> I'm glad to be getting to know you! As we went through your family history I noticed how hard it was for you stay present in the room when your feelings came up. Your parents numbed themselves with alcohol and diverted themselves with staying too busy to deal with (or should I say, not deal with) their emotions. It seems like you never got a chance to learn how to deal with emotion head on. We need to get you comfortable with feelings first and able to stay present as your most adult self. We'll start with little hand-weight-size emotions, then work up to the big ones. Then, you'll be able to stay in the room with your feelings when we go after the traumas. Does that make sense to you?
>
> I noticed that you've had a lot of trauma throughout your life. In my experience, if we start on the current ones, the old stuff comes up and takes us by surprise. If we nail the old ones first, the newer ones are usually easier. You've got about five big traumas that I see. (List them.) What if we process through them in order from the earliest to the most recent? (SDM). Or we could go after them starting with the least upsetting one and working up to the most distressing (SD phase model).
>
> I can't tell you exactly how many sessions your therapy will take, but I can make an educated guess. Unless we run into snags, I'm guessing 1 to 3 months to get up to bench-pressing the big feelings and one or two sessions each with the smaller traumas, and two to five sessions for the bigger ones. If I'm right, which I sometimes am, we're looking at 6 to 9 months to clear out most of the trauma.

A buy-in talk with a client with poor attachment, little affect tolerance, and a tremendous trauma history is different. You're dealing with a mixture of ego states, spacing out, somatic disruptions, confusion, and, often, terrible fear. You need to address the state changes that you noticed, without pathologizing the client. I name the parts using structural dissociation language (van der Hart et al., 2006).

> I see and feel how hard it was for you to go through your story. I noticed that big feelings came up and it was hard for you to talk. I want to show you how I make sense of what happens when you start spacing out or feeling really scared or mad. Then we'll talk about how to help.
>
> We all have different parts. We all can remember and feel emotions we've had before. When you've had a lot of trauma, you can be split into three kinds of parts. The apparently normal part of you is the part of you that goes to work, goes shopping, and connects with other people in day-to-day life. When something distressing happens outside of you, or if you remember something bad, your brain reflexively takes you to the emotional part. Your brain takes you right into the feelings and thoughts of the age when the trauma happened. It can take you into a mobilized part of you that's scared and wants to run, or mad and wants to fight, or scared and wants to grab onto someone. Or it takes you into an immobilized, shame-filled, shut-down depressed part. (Use examples from what you saw in the intake.) In your current life, you don't choose these states on purpose. But, back when you were a kid, they helped you deal with the abuse or neglect.
>
> Now, we'll work together so that you will have a choice about what states you're in. First, we'll build up your most grown-up part. I'll be right there with you, to help you get up to speed. When that grown-up part of you is ready to handle the old distressing emotions, we'll go after the old trauma and stop the automatic shifting to fight or flight or shut down. You'll get strong and you'll have a choice.
>
> I'll be honest: It's going to take a while. It took 18 years at home with that [fill in the blank] situation for you to develop those pieces of you. We have some great tools to work with. We'll use some guided imagery to help you calm down when the big feelings or flashbacks happen. We'll do some work that gets you able to feel without freaking out or spacing out. Other tools will help us get you

through the old trauma. I get the sense that you haven't gotten to feel much happiness. We can work together so that, eventually, you'll have the wiring to feel good. And then I'll help you learn how to operate in new ways with other people. Because there was so much abuse and so little support in your early life, I imagine at least 2 years of therapy, and probably more.

THERAPEUTIC RELATIONSHIP

In study after study, the client's sense of connection to the therapist was the highest predictor of therapeutic success. In 2006, the APA Presidential Task Force declared, "Psychological practice is, at root, an interpersonal relationship between psychologist and patient." Despite the number of whizbang trauma therapies you can conceptualize and do, if you can't connect with clients, you probably won't help them. Most trauma therapy trainings and books state the necessity for a strong therapeutic relationship but don't tell you how to make one. Others have attachment components built into the therapies themselves. These include but are not limited to Ogden's sensorimotor, Kitchur's strategic developmental model, and many of the psychodynamic-oriented trauma therapies, such as Fosha's accelerated experiential-dynamic psychotherapy and dyadic developmental psychotherapy.

How do you connect? Simple things help. Sit close, but not too close. Make, but do not demand eye contact. Respond! Respond to voice tonality and volume with your own voice. Respond to bodies: gestures, postures, tightening, relaxing. Respond to content. If it breaks your heart, you get to say that. If what happened to the client makes you mad, you get to be mad. Respond to affect. Don't tell someone it will be okay when it isn't. Do let clients know that you're in the room with them. Do let them know you notice what they feel. Many therapists can feel clients' affective and sometimes physical states in their own bodies. Using that information can build a strong bond. "I feel that anger/grief/fear in the room with us. Where are you feeling it in your body?" is a fair question. Read Diana Fosha's (2000) book, *The Transforming Power of Affect* for how to use language to respond to clients' distressing histories and affect.

If clients don't think and feel that you get them, know their strengths and vulnerabilities, and genuinely care about them, most won't go through the slog of facing their trauma and feeling horrible before they feel better. Some clients will make a good connection in a few minutes. Others may take months to begin to trust you. Your ability to connect is your best therapeutic tool.

The therapeutic relationship is especially important for clients who had early neglect or abuse, and the attending attachment deficits. For many of these clients, their attachment to you is what grows their right brain capacity for both attachment and affect tolerance.

Therapeutic Relationship and Attachment Resources

See the list in Chapter 25.

GUIDED IMAGERY AND RESOURCE INSTALLATION EXERCISES

With the rare trauma client with one adult-onset trauma, good attachment, and a supportive life, you do not need to do any imagery or resource installation before you start the trauma processing. Clients with poor attachment, poor affect regulation, or a currently distressing or disorganized life may or may not need the following state-changing exercises to prepare for the more distressing trauma work. The more pervasive the deprivation, trauma, and subsequent dissociation, the more connection to internal and external resources is necessary. Guided imagery is good for calming overwhelmed or highly symptomatic clients. Use it for symptom management until you can clear the trauma with effective techniques. Teach clients how to use imagery on their own, when they are distressed. If clients are religious, they may want to imagine that light or energy is coming from God or the heavens. If they're New Age, you may want to add chakras to the imagery. Utilize what is in the client's experience to guide your work. Pause between every sentence as your client responds. Track your client's every reaction. Don't move on until the client responds to the cues you just gave. Imagery work is not just reading scripts, it's a collaborative process. Let your client's response guide your timing and the direction of the work. Remember that you don't need to use these with stabilized clients. Remember that for some clients, going directly to clearing the trauma is the best stabilizing tool. Keep in mind that some exercises will work better with some clients than with others.

I'm throwing hypnotic boosts into these standard guided imagery exercises. As you read them, you'll be painlessly programming yourself to do hypnotic work.

Safe Place Exercise

As of October 2009, there were over 3 million entries on Google for "safe place exercise," and there's a good reason for it. "Safe place" is a part of the preparation phase of many psychotherapies. There are many versions. For clients who have had the experience of safety, here's what I do:

1. Have clients think about a place that's safe and brings a feeling of comfort. If they're having trouble thinking of a real place, have them make one up in their imagination.

2. Have them tell you what makes it safe.

3. Have them imagine being there, looking around, feeling the peacefulness. ("Hear the wind in the trees around the cabin, notice the quality of the light, and how snug and safe you feel, being there.") If they feel good and relaxed there, great. If they don't feel safe and relaxed, ask what needs to change.

4. Have them imagine visualizing the safe place when settling into bed or when distressed.

For clients who can't recall experiences of safety (many with secondary and nearly all with tertiary dissociation), the idea of safety may be distressing, so we change the name to "healing place" and build in deeper safety.

Imagine a healing place that is invisible to everyone but you. It can be on a seashore, in a forest, on a mountain, in the desert, or any place you want. To make it completely safe, it can even be off-planet. What did you pick? Great. What makes it healing? Wander around it and make sure that it suits you. You can change anything you want, because it's yours. No one else has a way in but you. Make sure there's a house or cabin (or in the case of polyfragmented DID clients, a mansion or condominium with a room for each full-blown part). Let's walk through the house, and notice how it's furnished, what kind of windows there are, what makes it secure, and what makes it healing. There's the kitchen. What's it like?

Make sure you have a magic refrigerator and magic cupboards with food that you adore, especially comfort food. There are no calories in the healing place. (For sexual abuse survivors) Let's explore the bedroom. How many locks are there on the inside of the door? How is the bed different from the bed that you had as a child? What makes it safe and healing? Let's walk the grounds. What do you see? Do you need an invisible containment field around the perimeter and overhead? Great, then do it. Figure out where you're going to put the healing pool. And when we work with inner children, what will they need here? (A swing set, a dog, a sandbox, toys, etc.) Make it so!

Later on, when we're doing the trauma clearing, if it ever gets too overwhelming, you can take a break and visit this healing place. When you're home and start feeling distress, or the flashbacks are bothering you, you can bring yourself here.

For clients with attachment issues: "If you could have any being you wanted, someone or something to watch over you, protect you, and always be ready to respond to you, 24/7, who or what you would want in the healing place?" People choose Jesus, Mary, a bodhisattva, Nana, the nurse-dog from Peter Pan, bears, the SuperNanny from television, angels, a generic good grandmother, or others. "Imagine that you get lonely. The angel is there to talk to, give hugs, or make hot chocolate. Imagine that you get scared. How will that angel protect you and comfort you? Stand guard with a sword? How about the comforting part? Hugs and jokes? Okay, make sure you get an angel with a sense of humor." Highly dissociated clients may have a room and a different protector for every part. Occasionally, clients with seemingly intractable insomnia begin to sleep by imagining themselves in their healing places, being watched over or held by their healing place attachment object.

Arc of Love

"Imagine everyone who loves or cares for you, where it hasn't gone bad, standing in an arc around you. It can be family, friends, professionals, dogs, and extraordinarily unselfish cats. Make contact with each person or critter, one at a time, through the eyes and through the heart, taking in the love and connection. Spend enough time with each one to really feel the love and totally take it in. Breathe it in, too. Let me know when you've gone around the whole arc." This exercise builds positive attachment and tolerance for positive affect. Don't do it with clients who have had no loving connections. If there is just one person, or one dog who loves them, do the exercise with that being. "Think of that moment when you walk in the door and are greeted by that good friend/excited dog. Feel that warmth coming toward you. Where do you feel that inside? Stay with that." Use this exercise as part of your assessment. People who do it easily tend to have good attachment and to tolerate positive affect. People who can't imagine any positive feeling coming toward them or from them may have big deficits in attachment and ability to tolerate positive affect, and a longer, harder healing road ahead of them.

Resource Installation

Roy Kiessling's (2005) extended resource development protocol enhances preexisting positive networks, then installs them, building new positive networks. It is one of many resourcing preparation phase techniques used in EMDR. This kind of resourcing is typically used with eye movements or other kinds of bilateral stimulation, but can be used without them.

The therapist says:

1. Think of a current problem.
2. Tell me what internal quality or strength you will need to surmount this problem.
3. Now think of a time when you used that quality effectively.
4. When you think of that time, what emotion do you feel right now? Where do you feel that in your body?
5. What word would go with that quality and your feeling when you think of it? (EMDR therapists would "install" that word with bilateral stimulation, BLS.)
6. Think of a recent time when it would have been helpful to be in touch with that internal resource and imagine using it (more BLS).
7. Great. Now think of using it successfully on the current problem (BLS).

8. And think of more times in the future when you could success-fully use that resource. (Go after specific problems or challenges with as many resources or qualities as you need.)

Container Exercise

Use containers for clients who have overwhelming emotions or physical sensations that are too much to process all at once (Kluft, 1988). The more dissociated the client, the easier it usually is to do this helpful dissociation exercise, though others can do it, too.

1. Imagine a container that's big enough and strong enough to hold all your feelings and distressing sensations. Describe it to me (anything from boxes and bottles to small-town water tanks or huge oil tanks).
2. Pour your distressing emotions into that container. Make sure you get them all in.
3. Are they in? Now find a way to lock that container up, so that nothing leaks out.
4. And let's put a tap or special airlock on your container so that together, at the right time, we can bring the sensations and emotions out a little at a time, for clearing.
5. If something triggers you into big, distressing feelings, or a flash-back, you can send all the feelings into the container. Imagine doing that, now.

Bringing in Light

What is your most healing color? Imagine this color moving through you from the top of your head all the way to your toes. Let this color permeate every organ, every cell, and every breath in your body. Breathe it in and out. In and out. That's right. Let it sweep every distressing feeling down through your feet. How far down do you have it now? Great! Keep breathing it down through your body. That's right. Is it at your feet yet? When it gets to your feet, let the light push all the distress and all the worry right out of you. That's right. Notice if there's any place in you that needs an extra dose of the healing light. Bring in more of that good light to that place. That's right.

Targeted Light Stream Technique

The light stream technique is a targeted version of bringing in light and is used by Stephen Levine (1991) for physical and emotional distress and by some EMDR therapists before trauma processing to take the edge off of traumatic distress or to help clients learn to identify and focus on sensation (Shapiro, 2001, pp. 244–245). I've brought in a bit of hypnotic technique in my version. This technique may permanently alter a distressing symptom or simply bring clients a temporary respite.

Do a body scan. Notice where you're holding tension and where you're relaxed. Bring a disturbing event to mind. (Specify the event.) Now scan through your body and notice where your body responds to that event. Where is it? What kind of feeling does it have? If that feeling had a shape, what would it be? And if it had a size, what would it be? What texture does it have? Does it have a color? Which of your favorite colors do you associate with healing? "Imagine your light coming through the top of your head and directing itself at that jagged, rough, red, enormous shape" (client's description). Imagine this light comes from the cosmos or God. The more you use, the more you have available. The light permeates the shape, resonating and vibrating in and around it. As it does, what is happening to the shape? What is happening to the color of it? Is the texture changing yet? Is the size changing yet? (If it's changing, continue.) What's happening to it now? Allow that part to completely heal. Any piece that isn't you can be swept out by the light. That's right. Now bring that good (blue) light through your entire body, filling your head, your shoulders, your torso, your arms, your pelvis, your legs, all the way down through your feet, moving the distress out. Feel that light in your breath. And notice if any part of your body needs an extra dose. That's right, allow the light in. Great!

Grounding Cord

As you sit on that couch, and notice your breathing, you can do a scan of your body, noticing where it feels easy and open and where it has tension. As you settle down into your body and breathe regularly, you notice how straightening your spine and sitting up allows more breath into your body. (The client sits more erect.) That's right. And you can imagine a cord moving down from the back of your head, down through the bones of your neck, and down through your spine.

When it reaches the bottom of your spine, notice how one strand of it goes straight down through the couch, through the floor, through the basement (modify for the building you're in) down, down, into the ground, and two other strands go down, down through your legs, around the corner of your knees, all the way through your feet and down, down through the building, into the ground. Feel these cords going down, down until they connect to the stone below the surface, rooting themselves in the strong, solid, dependable rock. That's right.

As you bring your attention to your body, you might notice how it's already responding to those cords that connect it deep, deep down to the ground. And you might be ready to let every distressing feeling in your mind and your body flow down those cords, down, down into the bedrock of the earth. Notice what feeling goes first and how fast it flows down that cord. Then notice what, as each distressing thought and feeling and burden flows down, your body feels like now. That's right. Let all the distress move down below the bedrock, dispersing through the stone, sinking toward the core of the earth, until it's so far away, so far away. That's right. And notice the good things you can pull up through those cords.

Can you feel the gravity that holds you to the couch? Can you remember that it's always been there and will always be there? And can you feel the deep calm of the earth begin to flow up the cords, up, up through your feet, up, up through your spine, filling your body with deep calm, grounding your body with a sense of connection to the earth, the entire planet supporting you, holding you, there for you? And every time you remember to feel your connection, you will feel the support of this earth. (At these points, as appropriate, I'll add a reference to "God's earth," "feeling yourself held in the hand of the Goddess," "feeling connected to every living being," or whatever works for the person in front of me.) And every time you don't remember to feel the connection, parts of you will know that the earth is there, supporting you. (Covering all the bases.) As you breathe, you might imagine breathing in the ground-

edness through the bottom of your feet and through that cord connected to your spine and breathing out the same way. Breathing in
(in time with the client's breath) and out. In and out. That's right.
And every time you breathe, part of you will know that you're connected to the best parts of the earth, and held, by its gravity, to all
that is good. (Two posthypnotic suggestions:) And when you leave
here, and you're at home and at work and anyplace you go and
walking between places you go to, you can often remember to notice that cord from your spine and those cords from your feet sink
deeply, deeply into the surface of the planet, grounding you, releas-
ing distress, and bringing you the support of gravity and connection
to the whole earth. And if something distresses you, your body may
automatically know that it can feel these cords connecting it to the
healing, grounding capacity of the earth, and you can automatically
find the strength of the earth enhancing your own strength to deal
with whatever problems and whatever feelings arise in your life.

CLINICAL WRAP-UP

Remember that most guided imagery exercises offer a respite from
trauma but don't take it away. While they can be valuable tools for
preparation and throughout the therapy, they are not a substitute for
clearing the trauma. Some therapists are overcautious and waste valuable sessions doing every possible ego-strengthening and body-calming
technique when they could have launched into trauma processing.
Check inside with your own fear to see if it's the client's need or yours
that keeps you in the preparation phase when it's time to move on to
trauma processing. When your client has a supportive family, good
attachment, a relaxed temperament, affect tolerance, a few adult-
onset traumas, and a good connection with you, you can skip these
exercises.

Part III

TRAUMA TREATMENTS

CHAPTER FIVE

Mindfulness

If, according to Dan Siegel (2007), "the mind can be defined as an embodied and relational process that regulates the flow of energy and information," (p. 111) then mindfulness might be the conscious awareness and control of those flows. The brain handles all kinds of tasks without direct intervention from the mind. It regulates hormonal output, heart rate, circadian rhythms, and hundreds of other systems. It also registers potential threats (some of which are echoes of historical threats) and responds before the mind has time to get online and think about the situation. Bringing the resources of the mind to the reflexes of the body and brain allows us to control and sometimes vanquish reflexive trauma responses.

The ultimate goals of any trauma therapy are that clients be in the present with no intrusion from past distressing events, no fear of that intrusion or their own affect, and the ability to function and to relate well to themselves and others. Mindfulness supports all these goals.

Near the beginning of therapy, until you have a chance to clear the trauma, you can teach mindfulness as a way to cope with PTSD and other trauma symptoms. In the long run, it can work as a trauma treatment. A woman at a meditation retreat who had a horrific abuse history spoke about how meditation had helped her. She said, "After 5 years of meditation, I sat drinking my coffee in the breakfast nook, and for the first time, I saw the wall across from me, and only the wall. I felt only sensations and emotions that went with sitting in my breakfast nook, no abuse memories. Then I felt tremendous relief. I was finally here, in the present!"

MEDITATION

The first task of mindfulness is presence. Luckily, there are many paths to "be here now." Some meditation practices teach attention to a single point of consciousness. As you focus on your breath or your walking stride or a mantra or an image, you notice what else your mind throws at you, then, over and over, go back to your object of focus. I tell clients, "It strengthens the muscles in your brain, allowing them to develop the ability to direct your brain. It also allows you to take a step back from what you're going through and just notice the flashbacks, weird old sensations, and bad thoughts go by."

For the skeptical, I quote research: "Sarah Lazar and colleagues at the Massachusetts General Hospital completed an fMRI imaging study of 20 people engaged in meditation involving sustained mindful attention to internal and external sensory stimuli and nonjudgmental awareness of present-moment stimuli without cognitive elaboration. They found that brain regions associated with attention, interoception, and sensory processing were thicker in meditation participants than matched controls, including the prefrontal cortex and right anterior insula" (van der Kolk, 2006, p. 288).

There have been at least two movies about Vipassana (a form of mindfulness meditation) in prisons: *Doing Time, Doing Vipassana* (Menahemi & Ariel, 1997) and *The Dhamma Brothers* (Phillips & Stein, 2008). In the latter, prisoners in an Alabama maximum security prison go through a 10-day meditation retreat. Many said that it was the hardest thing they ever did, and spoke about learning to sit with the memories and emotions connected to lifelong trauma, including the murders they committed. As they learned to be present with their own experience, they learned affect tolerance, acceptance, and began to grow the ability to be here and now. Their relationships changed as they learned to observe their affect and automatic responses and make good choices in their interactions with each other. They developed mindfulness and presence in 10 days of intensive practice. As they brought meditation into their daily lives, they continued to heal from trauma, get present, and get along (Stein, 2008).

Mindfulness Meditation Exercise (Internal Focus)

The first time I start with a warning: "This exercise works well for a lot of people. Once in a while it brings up big distressing feelings. If that happens, let me know, and we'll do something with them."

> Put your feet on the floor. Sit comfortably straight in that chair. Let your arms rest. As you sit there, I'm not asking you to change anything but your awareness. Start with noticing your breath. Notice it filling your lungs and notice your belly rise and fall with each breath. That's right. Breathing in . . . breathing out . . . breathing in . . . breathing out . . . (30 seconds.) . . . Now notice it's more complicated than that. Right after you breathe out, notice that you pause for a short moment before the next breath. Do you notice that? Good. Now notice the little pause before you breathe out again. Watch yourself breathing out, the pause, breathing in, and the pause. Go with that on your own for a few minutes. . . . Now notice what else floats through your awareness. Images? Thoughts? Other body sensations? Memories? That's all fine and absolutely normal. Every time you notice your mind doing what it likes to do, thinking, bring your attention back to your breath. You will do this maybe a few hundred times each time you meditate, in your early meditation practice, and maybe only a hundred, when you've gotten really good at it. Breathing out. Pause. Breathing in. Pause. Breathing out. That's right. . . . And as you notice what thoughts and sensations and feelings float by in the sea of your awareness, notice that you'll become able to just notice them, without as much identification. It's a thought. Okay. It's a feeling. Okay. It's an image. Okay. Breathing out, noticing the pause, breathing in, pause, breathing and noticing.

If clients can tolerate this mindfulness practice, I ask them to try it for 10 minutes each day, and report back. If they love it, I suggest twice a day. And if at the next session, they actually did the practice at home, I might suggest 20 minutes each day. If they become regular meditators, we can use their practice as an immediate self-regulation device: "Whoa, John, it looks like you're starting to panic while you're remembering the shooting. Right now, bring your attention back to your breath. Breathing in, breathing out. Notice the pauses at each end? Good, keep noticing your breath. . . . Good, you're calmer. Let's go at this one more slowly, so you can stay in the room while we clear it out."

EXTERNALLY FOCUSED PRESENCE

In my experience, two kinds of clients can't tolerate internally focused exercises. Both constitutionally anxious people and those with huge bodily PTSD reactions may regard their bodies as bad neighborhoods to be avoided at all costs. After all, bodies are where those overwhelming feelings live. These clients initially can bring their foci outside their bodies to notice what's around them.

Three Things

Thom Negri (personal communication, 1984) taught me to help immediately dissociative or panicked people to bring their attention into the room. The exercise goes like this: "Look around the room, and tell me three things that are red. Now, three things that are blue. Now, tell me three sounds you hear. Now, three textures you can see or feel. Now, if it feels safe, look into my eyes and notice what you see."

We practice this technique in sessions when clients are flooded and either too mobilized or immobilized. I tell them to use it at home, "when you're either freaking out or spacing out, to bring yourself back to the room."

Beauty Awareness

I invented an externally focused technique: beauty awareness. People do it when they're not completely panicked or shut down, but getting that way. It goes like this: "Look around you, and notice anything that pleases your eye. Check out the pictures in the room, the view out the window, the places where two walls meet the ceiling and the light falls differently on each surface. Pick the thing that draws you the most, and keep your attention right there. (After about a minute) What do you notice now? Now bring your attention to another object or surface that catches your eye. Stay with that awhile, and then tell me what you notice." Most people tell me that they feel calmer. Some begin to smile and tell me that it makes them happy.

People who never do other homework often do this exercise. They report that they begin to seek out beauty and to notice and feel present in the current time and place more often. It works especially well with constitutionally anxious people. One client with obsessive-compulsive disorder said that she was starting to replace her ruminations with "beauty breaks." Clients with disorders of extreme stress or DID may have different reactions. One said, "I was so busy worrying about what was going to happen next, I didn't know it was okay for me to notice the good things around. This is great!" The other said, "I can't do this. It's not safe not to be hyperalert all the time. If I try to do it, I feel too scared." The first client knows he's here now. The second is more dissociative and hasn't gotten enough of himself present for this exercise to work.

YOGA

Bessel van der Kolk, the famous trauma researcher, was so impressed with his 2006 research on the effects of yoga on his traumatized clients that he set up yoga classes in his clinic. From a 2007 *Yoga Journal* article, D. K. Wills reports: "[Van der Kolk] says, 'Yoga reestablishes the sense of time. You notice how things change and flow inside your body.' Learning relaxation and breathing techniques helps PTSD patients calm themselves down when they sense that a flashback or panic attack is coming. And yoga's emphasis on self-acceptance is important for victims of sexual assault, many of whom hate their bodies."

Walter Reed Army Medical Center holds yoga classes for active-duty soldiers with PTSD. Preliminary research shows that it alleviates some of the symptoms. Wills (2007) cites several other studies of positive results for veterans and soldiers with PTSD. Michelle Ma (2009), who works for my local paper, the *Seattle Times*, wrote about local Iraq War veterans doing meditation and yoga at the Seattle VA hospital. I tracked down Dr. David Kearney to find out about his program.

Dr. Kearney, a physician, researcher, and professor at the University of Washington, also works at the Seattle VA. Pursuing his own mindfulness practice, he studied with Jon Kabat-Zinn. He bases his mindfulness-based stress reduction (MBSR) program on Kabat-Zinn's (1990) recommendations in his useful book, *Full Catastrophe Living*. Hundreds of veterans have cycled through the 8-week program since 2007. Through mindfulness training, they strive to pay attention to the present moment without judgment. Each session is 2½ hours long, including at least 45 minutes of discussion of mindfulness issues. Between weeks 6 and 7, they gather on Saturday for 7 hours of silent practice. In the first class, they spend 5 minutes eating one raisin and are asked to keep their attention on only the sensations of eating that raisin. "This brings home to them that their minds are often on automatic pilot." In week 2, they learn Kabat-Zinn's comprehensive body scan, "moving their attention systematically from one place in the body to the next." In week 3, it's mindful movement, yoga. They practice awareness of breath and different forms of meditation, including walking meditation.

Most of the vets in the program are in psychotherapy. Very few drop out of the group. After the 8 weeks, many veterans continue in a "continuity" peer sitting group. Many report, during the 8 weeks and in follow-up, that the mindfulness practice has lessened their avoidance of traumatic material, reshaped their patterns of vigilance, and lessened their reexperiencing of the traumatic events. They feel less angry and are angry less often. They get along better with other people. Many have commented that their family members are telling them how much easier they are to be around. Dr. Kearney received a 2008 pilot grant from the Puget Sound Partners of Global Health (which includes the Gates Foundation) to study the efficacy of his program. Half of the subjects are doing his MBSR group, and half are doing treatment as usual, cognitive behavior therapy, prolonged exposure, and medication. He says that his preliminary results are promising.

MARTIAL ARTS

Some martial arts can be stress-reducing and mindfulness inducing, especially tai chi, qigong, and aikido. People, especially male people, who would never do meditation, yoga, or psychotherapy, might do martial arts. Many martial arts classes are slanted toward self-protection. Some, such as model mugging, are for protection against sexual assault. Assault survivors often take these classes, learning awareness, grounding, and their own strength, while working through the reflexive ventral vagal freeze and dorsal vagal shutdown response that went with the initial assault or sexual abuse. Others are more meditative. All bring clients into their bodies, increasing affect tolerance and presence.

MINDFULNESS OF THE THERAPIST

Dan Siegel (2009) uses an acronym, PARTTTT, to explain that when therapists are fully

Present we can

Attune to the client or others and

Resonate with others and develop

Trust, which is important because it activates the smart ventral vagus so the social engagement system turns on, so that we can

Track what's going on in moment-to-moment experience, which allows the

Truth to come out and creates

Transformation and healing

We therapists, when therapeutically attuned, reflexively absorb, mirror, and often feel what our clients are experiencing. We must develop practices that keep us in the room and in ourselves when a client is either emoting or dissociating. Mindfulness allows us to notice our minds and mental and emotional states as they change throughout our sessions. It allows us to think, "I'm spacing out. Is my client dissociating again?" "Why am I feeling angry? I wasn't when I walked in the room. I wonder if it's this client's disowned anger? I'll ask her. 'Janet, is there another feeling under that sadness?' Bingo! It's anger."

When I'm doing clinical consultation, when therapists tell me that they're feeling hopeless about a case, I ask them to go inside and check if it's the client's hopelessness or theirs. Therapists can develop mindfulness the old fashioned ways, through meditation or yoga. We can pursue our own therapy, so that we know when our issues and affects are mobilized by our clients' issues and affects. A good consultant can be a therapeutic mindfulness coach. The goal of therapeutic mindfulness is bringing full attention to our clients, while monitoring our own responses.

CLINICAL WRAP-UP

Meditation instruction is readily available through books, classes, audio materials, and retreats. Meditation, yoga, and martial arts classes are ubiquitous. The classes can be a source of social support. People can practice meditation and yoga, tai chi and qigong on their own. The effects are cumulative, leading to more focused attention, more affect tolerance, and mindfulness. It is possible for some people to clear trauma symptoms on their own with these techniques. All of these modalities help keep the left brain and the adult, human, mindful brain online during stressful events. Meditation, yoga, and martial arts instruction are not as culturally stigmatized as psychotherapy. Meditators and yoga practitioners bring their focus, affect tolerance, and experience of dual attention to psychotherapy, often advancing faster than other clients, regardless of therapy modality.

However, most meditation and yoga instructors are not equipped to deal with full-blown PTSD or other dissociative symptoms. Many traumatized people experience flashbacks during meditation or yoga postures that drive them away from the techniques. Some of these people will doggedly stay with their modality, adding a new layer of dissociation as they practice. For most trauma sufferers, mindfulness, while a wonderful tool, isn't enough for them to completely move through their dissociative symptoms. A combination of mindfulness practice and psychotherapy is often the best medicine for trauma survivors, especially those with complex trauma histories.

MINDFULNESS MATERIALS

About What's Been Done

Stephen Cope's anthology, *Will Yoga and Meditation Really Change My Life: Personal Stories from 25 of North America's Leading Teachers* (Kripalu Center for Yoga and Health, 2003).

Daniel Siegel's comprehensive book, *The Mindful Brain: Reflection and Attunement in the Cultivation of Well-Being* (Norton, 2007).

Jenny Stein, *Letters from the Dhamma Brothers: Meditation Behind Bars* (Pariyatti Press, 2008).

The movie *Doing Time, Doing Vipassana* (Menahemi, A., & Ariel, E., Karuna Films, 1997).

The movie *The Dhamma Brothers* (Phillips, P., & Stein, A. M., Freedom Behind Bars Productions, 2008).

And many, many Web sites and research articles, for which you can search.

About How to Do It

Jack Kornfield, *Meditation for Beginners* (Sounds True, 2004).

Jon Kabat-Zinn, *Mindfulness for Beginners* (audio CD). Also get his book, *Full Catastrophe Living: Using the Wisdom of Your Body and Mind to Face Stress, Pain, and Illness* (Dell, 1990).

Dan Siegel, *Mindsight: The New Science of Personal Transformation* (Bantam, 2010).

There's even a *Meditation for Dummies* by Stephan Bodian and Dean Ornish (Wiley, 2006).

My favorite mindfulness books are by Thich Nhat Hahn, a Vietnamese monk. For beginners, *The Miracle of Mindfulness* (Beacon Press, 1975). More specifically for trauma, *Taming the Tiger Within: Meditations on Transforming Difficult Emotions* (Penguin Books, 2005).

CHAPTER SIX

Psychodynamic Therapies

Each of the many dynamic therapies has its own theory and focus of function. I'll touch on only a few of the modern dynamically influenced psychotherapies: dyadic developmental psychotherapy (DDP), accelerated empathetic therapy (AET), attachment-based intensive short-term dynamic psychotherapy (AB/ISTDP), and accelerated experiential-dynamic psychotherapy (AEDP). There isn't room enough to describe the immense contributions of Sigmund Freud (1856–1939) and his daughter Anna Freud (1895–1982) that form the basis of psychodynamic therapies. Diana Fosha's writings give substance to the short-term dynamic therapy psychotherapy (STDP) section.

Dynamic therapies hold the therapist-client relationship as central to the therapeutic process. Traditional psychoanalysis cautions that a therapist must hold a neutral position, so as not to interfere with the client's process, and to give clients a clean surface on which to project. Melanie Klein (1882–1960), trained by Freud, brought ideas of attachment and projective identification to the dynamic table. She developed object relations theory, which became the second leg of the tripod of analytic thought. Her object relations work was advanced through Donald Winnicott (1896–1971) and many others. Short-Term Dynamic Psychotherapy (STDP), as developed by Davanloo (1980), uses the relationship to hammer quickly through defenses. Diana Fosha (2000), in her Accelerated Experiential Dynamic Psychotherapy (AEDP), and Robert Neborsky's (2006) Attachment-Based Intensive Short Term Dynamic Therapy (AB/ISTDP) marry Winnicott's and newer attachment techniques with Davanloo's STDP to do deep, fast, supportive work.

Traditionally, dynamic therapies were interested in the psychic defenses and in bringing the unconscious mind to consciousness and to the clients' understanding of events and themselves. Traditional analysis delves deeply into meaning. Looking at analytic therapy through the structural dissociation lens (Chapter 3), the focus would be on the EPs and the processes that hold the EP separate from the ANP. Some older dynamic models, based on Anna Freud's theories, have their own ego state configurations, including the infantile, emotional id that wants what it wants; the internalized family and cultural influences of the ego, which is the intermediary between the id and the outside world; and the adult, functional, reasoning superego.

Judith Chertoff (1998) writes that a traditional psychodynamic therapy for trauma involves "1) assessing the impact of trauma on the patient's ego defensive functioning and 2) elucidating the dynamic meaning of both the patient's presenting symptoms and the traumatic events that precipitated them" (p. 35). The therapist engages the reasoning superego, while discussing the trauma and its impacts on the client's system, strengthening the superego, slowly dismantling the trauma-based defenses, and bringing understanding, affect tolerance, and calm to the system. The training to learn the concepts and techniques of doing traditional psychodynamic therapy takes years, and I can't write much more about it here without getting well beyond the scope of this book.

Chertoff (1998) paraphrases Anna Freud (1967), who wrote that five factors influence the outcome of trauma:

1. The nature and intensity of the trauma

2. Sensitization due to prior trauma

3. Hereditary and congenital factors that affect the level of defensive functioning (there's temperament again)

4. Chronological age and developmental stage at the time of the trauma

5. Environment at the time of trauma

Chertoff offers a sixth factor from McFarlane and Yehuda (1996): preexisting personality. "Character traits, more fully consolidated by adulthood, further affect the outcome of adult trauma, leaving some individuals more susceptible to protracted PTSD reactions than others" (p. 43). These factors make sense in any therapy conceptualization.

Dyadic Developmental Psychotherapy

DDP is a family therapy based on attachment theory, an integration of several methods that have a strong evidence base. According to Dan Hughes and Arthur Becker-Weidman (2008),

> [DDP] was originally developed to treat children with disorders of attachment. . . . It has since been more broadly used to help families with a variety of difficulties, including complex trauma. . . . DDP has as its core, or central therapeutic mechanism for treatment success, the maintenance of a contingent, collaborative, sensitive, reflective and affectively attuned relationship between therapist and child, between caregiver and child, and between therapist and caregiver. DDP focuses on and relies upon the intersubjective sharing and joint development and organization of emotional experience. (p. 329)

Hughes and Becker-Weidman speak about intersubjectivity, wherein the parent and child experience themselves as having an impact on the experience of the other. "For example, children experience themselves as being delightful, lovable and clever whenever their parents experience them as manifesting those characteristics. In a similar way, the parents experience themselves as being capable and caring whenever their children experience them as manifesting those traits" (p. 330).

DDP basic principles include the importance of parents' and therapists' good attachment capacity and ability to provide positive intersubjective experiences for children. It's all about attunement. It includes good acronyms: PACE—the therapist sets a healing pace for treatment by being **p**layful, **a**ccepting, **c**urious, and **e**mpathetic; and PLACE—the parent creates a healing environment by being **p**layful, **l**oving, **a**ccepting, **c**urious, and **e**mpathetic. DDP emphasizes repair of misattunements and conflicts, which helps with affect regulation and teaches that conflict doesn't necessarily lead to abandonment or abuse.

In DDP, both children and parents are involved with the process. Both learn to attune, to make repair, to giggle together, and hold the sadness and pain of life. The parents learn to be therapeutic by being well-connected. The therapy with the children looks informal, with lots of back and forth, co-relating of stories, and cocreation of right-now reality. Resistance is handled with curiosity. Trauma is handled together, with the therapist giving words to the old experience. Parents are taught how to touch their kids to provide solace, engagement, and containment. And parents are assessed for attachability.

It's a great therapy for reactive attachment, for trauma, and for kids with any attachment disruptions. In my experience, the principles work with adults, too. It's part of how I work with trauma, tying inter-subjective experience, room for positive and negative affect, with targeted EMDR, Brainspotting, and ego state strategies thrown into the mix.

SHORT-TERM DYNAMIC PSYCHOTHERAPY

Intensive short-term dynamic psychotherapy (ISTDP) is the most intense therapy I've ever seen on video. ISTDP therapists relentlessly hammer at defenses while maintaining safety and trust. Clients drop their defenses, acknowledge, feel and express emotions, and then make sense of it all, FAST! According to Diana Fosha in *The Trans-forming Power of Affect*, all STDPs consider "the experiential compo-nent . . . the experience of previously unbearable affect in the here and now of the patient-therapist relationship, as the key agent of the thera-peutic change. . . . STDPs are united in the search for the most effec-tive, efficient and comprehensive therapeutic methods for maximizing affective experiences and minimizing the impact of defensiveness and anxiety" (2000, p. 314). Fosha explains the common ground of the ex-periential STDPs (pp. 318–321):

1. Schematicized psychodynamic constructs of how core emotional experiences and defense mechanisms are structured.

2. Rapid structuring of clinical material.

3. Trial therapy: "the therapist enters the relationship with the pa-tient ready for active dynamic interaction from the get-go."

4. Patient capacity for dynamic interaction as a major selection cri-terion. (This therapy couldn't work with a person with functional disturbances, an inability to connect, or too much dissociation.)

5. Active engagement of the patient as partner in the treatment endeavor.

6. Setting a termination date at the beginning of the treatment, to keep the client focused and on track.

7. Use of explicit criteria for assessment of fluctuations in depth of unconscious communication and rapport. "[T]he therapist monitors the patient's response to each intervention, paying particular attention to qualitative shifts in the depth of the unconscious communication and fluctuations in rapport." Which, in turn, becomes grist for the therapeutic mill. The "therapist [constantly] refines interventions according to the patient's responses."

8. Using the focus to guide selective therapeutic responding. The psychodynamic formulation, the focus, based on "dynamic exploration of the patient's past, present, and now also transferential conflicts . . . guided by shifts in the level of rapport and depth of unconscious communication."

9. "The use of interpretations to bring into consciousness and enable the patient to experience his emotions" (Malan, 1976, p. 259). These interpretations are dynamic in more ways than one. They take no prisoners and allow no defense. They move the client and the therapy forward, pronto. Many of the interpretations aim at uncovering the client's rage and sadistic impulses, especially the rage and destructive urges toward the self.

Davanloo's ISTDP is about intense, visceral access to feelings and body awareness. Defenses are considered to include verbal mannerisms, avoidance of eye contact, body stances, and vocal qualities. He uses challenge and pressure to clarify what's happening within the client and in the therapy interaction. He and his adherents demand straightforward communication and total engagement: "Insight is formally and unequivocally replaced by visceral experience as the sought-for catalytic agent. The actual here-and-now experience and expression of previously unconscious feelings and impulses within the transference relationship is the aim of Davanloo's technique" (Fosha, 2000, p. 328). (Compare this with Chapter 10 on somatic therapies.)

Fosha finds some problems with ISTDP. First, it makes such demands on therapists that few can do it. She says it's suited more to lawyers than therapists. We clinicians often aren't aggressive enough. And "many patients are similarly overwhelmed and find it difficult to respond to ISTDP. Finally, the conceptualization of all psychopathology as motivated by self-destructive aims, actually applies to only a limited number of patients" (2000, p. 330).

ACCELERATED EMPATHETIC THERAPY

AET looks like the opposite of ISTDP, though it uses some of the same techniques. Instead of rage, grief is the main event. "The mourning process becomes the main pathway to healing" (Fosha, 2000, p. 333). Instead of hammering, the AET therapist uses safety and quieter emotional engagement. The therapist uses "corrective emotional experiences" to do an end run around defenses. Empathy and showing compassion are key. Defenses are reframed and appreciated as having been necessary (which is useful in any therapy). The therapist's self-disclosure is used to short-circuit the patient's defensiveness and to demonstrate the therapist's willingness to share difficult, intense affective experiences with the patient.

Fosha finds some problems with AET. It "remains a one-stance, one-etiology, one-pathway-to-change treatment model" (p. 334): just about grief; sometimes too much about the therapist; and too intrapsychically focused.

ACCELERATED EXPERIENTIAL-DYNAMIC PSYCHOTHERAPY

Both Robert Neborsky and Diana Fosha took the ISTDP work of Malan and Davanloo and brought in conscious attachment components. Neborsky married his work to the attachment research of Mary Main and Eric Hesse to create Attachment Based Intensive Short Term Dynamic Psychotherapy AB/ISTDP. Fosha developed AEDP, which attempts to solve some of the problems of the other STDPs. It's more flexible, with a more general focus that encompasses different dynamics and core affects and is usable by a wider range of clinicians and clients. According to Fosha, "the common underlying factor is the visceral experience of affect in the context of an emotionally engaged dyadic relationship as a path to transformation. . . . [It's an] affect centered model of relational psychodynamics . . . rooted in the change-oriented work of attachment theorists and clinical developmentalists" (2000, p. 336). It's about affective competence. The therapist provides an affect-facilitative environment: safe and fear-free. It's healing centered rather than about pathology, going toward an "expanded realm of core affective phenomena . . . that includes self and relational affective experiences, as well as the core state" (p. 337). AEDP favors experience over traditional dynamic understanding. Therapists are empathetic and strive for affect facilitation, radically accepting the client "as he is now and [using] focused efforts to help him to become as deeply himself as he can." It's permissible, as an AEDP therapist, to focus on positive affects, to rejoice at breakthroughs or good news as well as grief, shame, and rage. AEDP celebrates joy and therapists are encouraged to share their affective responses to all of clients' experiences and emotions.

One of my favorite components of AEDP is its use of attachment-based language to facilitate the therapeutic relationship and the clients' affective awareness. I think that Fosha brings the left-brain cognitive awareness to the right-brain affective and physical experience when she asks questions like, "What's it like to know how happy I am to see you so alive?" "What's it like to feel that anger and know that it's justified and know that I know it's justified?" "What's it like to express that feeling after so many years of holding it back and to have me witness it with support?"

How Do STDPs Work With Trauma?

In a 5-day AEDP intensive class, I watched at least 10 hours of videos of Diana Fosha working with her clients. The trauma therapists sat in a group up front and told each other what Fosha was doing, through our lenses. What did we see? Fosha showed presence. She watched her clients like a hawk, responding to every breath, twitch, statement, and movement. She kept her clients right at the edge of their tolerance, neither hyperaroused (too agitated) nor hypoaroused (too quiet). She and the clients were consistently engaged, with each other and with the material. She masterfully used language that brought the client to present experiences of self, affect, and the supportive presence of the therapist. Sometimes she did a form of ego state work: "What was that little girl feeling back then? What are you feeling about her?" When she and the clients talked about traumatic events (exposure), the constant mindfulness of the relationship between them and the awareness of the body sensations and the shifting affects were dual attentions that kept the clients present in the room, feeling and tolerating affect, until the affects were felt, completed, and integrated. One us of said, "It's just like EMDR, with the relationship as the dual attention." We all agreed. At the end of each session, Diana and her clients discussed the meaning of the work and the emotions they felt about the work and each other.

AEDP, as practiced by Fosha, its inventor, is gorgeous work. It goes quickly. The clients feel good about the work and about themselves. The trauma clears as readily as with any therapy I've seen. The EP states integrate with the ANP to create a healed, happier, posttraumatized person with a broader range of affect and self-acceptance, free of PTSD symptoms.

CLINICAL WRAP-UP

These new dynamically informed therapies emphasize both the therapeutic relationship and affect, major components of healing trauma. The short-term dynamic therapies solve the problems of time and expense that have prohibited many people from partaking in traditional, long-term psychodynamic treatments. Good dynamic practitioners, whether in DDP, STDPs, or myriad others, are taught how to attune with and respond to clients' affect, narrative, and state shifts. Trauma therapists of any stripe can benefit from a grounding in newer dynamic approaches to the therapeutic relationship.

Traditional dynamic therapies often focus on intrapsychic phenomena to the exclusion of here-and-now trauma recovery. Some of the newer STDPs might be too focused on one affect (anger or grief) to take on the myriad emotions that go with trauma.

RESOURCES

Diana Fosha, *The Transforming Power of Affect: A Model for Accelerated Change* (Basic Books, 2000). No matter what kind of therapy you do, if you read this book, you'll do it better. Great information about attachment, affect, and how to do good therapy.

Marion Solomon and Daniel Siegel's *Healing Trauma* (2006) has chapters by Fosha, Neborsky, and many of the researchers and therapists in trauma therapy. Many of the chapters are dense. All are packed with information and give you strong descriptions of two STDPs.

Michael Alpert and Robert Neborsky, *Short Term Therapy for Long Term Change* (Norton, 2001).

The AEDP Institute and Diana Fosha's Web site, classes, practitioner list, and more, http://www.aedpinstitute.com/

Robert Neborsky's Web site, http://home.pacbell.net/highbid/ISTDP .html

Arthur Becker-Weidman's DDP Web site, with training DVDs and other resources, http://www.center4familydevelop.com/

The main DDP Web site, http://www.danielhughes.org/

There are analytic training programs in nearly every major U.S. city, especially in the Northeast. Hundreds of books, journals, and continuing education programs are available. Because the newer dyadic and short-term forms are not as widespread, you might have to travel for the training. In Southern California, you can study with Neborsky. In New York, you can study with Fosha. There are STDP enclaves in many cities. If you organize training in your town, you can probably entice an expert to teach the class.

CHAPTER SEVEN

Exposure Therapies

Exposure therapy (EX) is the name for a group of behavioral therapies in which anxious or traumatized clients are confronted either imaginally or in vivo with the thing or event they would most like to avoid. EX is often categorized as a cognitive behavior therapy, but I see the more simple EX therapies as working differently. Typically, therapists and clients make an anxiety hierarchy, a list of what the client fears. Some therapies start with the most distressing event, some with a moderately distressing event. Clients are exposed to the frightening stimulus until they feel less anxious or show fewer symptoms. When the therapy is successful, clients show less avoidance and fewer PTSD symptoms.

Exposure is a component of nearly all trauma therapies. Among other things, exposure confronts avoidance, one of the criteria of the PTSD diagnosis in the *DSM-IV*:

> Persistent avoidance of stimuli associated with the trauma and numbing of general responsiveness (not present before the trauma), as indicated by three (or more) of the following: (1) efforts to avoid thoughts, feelings, or conversations associated with the trauma; (2) efforts to avoid activities, places, or people that arouse recollections of the trauma; (3) inability to recall an important aspect of the trauma. (American Psychiatric Association, 2000, p. 468)

Remember how the structural dissociation model segregates the daily activity ANP from the traumatized parts of the EP? Our brains appear to use our own endogenous opiate system to help us not feel pain, including the pain of traumatic experience (Lanius, 2002, 2003, 2005; Lanius et al., 2002). And when we avoid thinking about things that distress us, like trauma, our brains give us feel-good drugs for our avoidance (Goleman, 1985). (This is the basis of procrastination, but that's another book.) Many trauma survivors make conscious decisions to avoid trauma triggers. "Since my rape, I never want to see a movie where a woman is in danger." "I never go by that corner, since the car accident." But our opiate and endorphin systems create their own unconscious reinforcement for staying away from or thinking about traumatic material.

As trauma therapists, it's our job to find a way around this avoidance reflex. If clients have good affect tolerance, good enough attachment to accept therapeutic support, and strong mindful senses of the here and now, simple exposure exercises can help teach their brains that the trauma is over, they're here, and there's nothing to avoid. If clients can't tolerate or regulate their affect and can't stay present during the therapy, simple exposure therapy can sometimes exacerbate symptoms, creating long horrible flashbacks that can drive clients out of therapy, increase substance use, or stimulate suicidal thoughts or actions.

Behaviorism supplies the ideas behind EX. In EX thinking, flashbacks and distressing arousal are maintained by classical conditioning. In this modality, avoidance, substance abuse, and dissociation are conditioned ways to manage trauma. Rothbaum, Meadows, Resick, and Foy (2000) explain Foa and Kozak's (1986) emotional processing theory, which "holds that PTSD emerges due to a development of a pathological fear structure concerning the traumatic event. . . . Any information associated with the trauma activates the fear structure." They say that therapists must activate the fear structure and "provide new information that is incompatible with existing compatible elements . . . thus integrating corrective information and modifying the pathological elements of the trauma memory" (p. 61).

There are many kinds of EX. Wolpe (1958) taught his clients how to relax deeply, then elicited the trauma response, then took them back to the relaxed state, then the trauma, then more relaxation. He called his theory reciprocal inhibition, with the idea that if you're relaxed, you can't be anxious. Later, you'll see this kind of pendulation between emotional states in EMDR, David Grand's Brainspotting work, Peter Levine's somatic experiencing, and other modalities.

PROLONGED EXPOSURE

Some EX techniques skip the relaxation and go straight for the trauma, trying to elicit distress in order to learn to tolerate it. Edna Foa's prolonged exposure elicits the trauma imaginally or directly with a physical trigger (Foa, Hembree, & Rothbaum, 2007). Clients make a tape of their trauma event in each therapy session, and then go home and listen to the tape every day. They also choose a previously avoided activity to do each day. Someone with PTSD from a car accident might listen to their tape about the accident, then do the following:

1. Spend time sitting in the car

2. Later, sit in the car and turn on the ignition

3. Sit in the car with the motor running for 5 minutes

4. Later, drive down the driveway

5. Then later, down the street

6. Then later, drive on the highway on which the accident occurred

Exposure Resources

Edna Foa, E. A. Hembree, and B. O. Rothbaum, *Prolonged Exposure Therapy for PTSD: Emotional Processing of Traumatic Experiences Therapist Guide* (Oxford University Press, 2007).

Edna Foa, Kelly Chrestman, and Eva Gilboa-Schectman, *Prolonged Exposure Therapy for Adolescents with PTSD: Emotional Processing of Traumatic Experiences, Therapist Guide* (Oxford University Press, 2008).

VIRTUAL REALITY

Some therapists use virtual reality exposure, gradually exposing clients to the sights and sounds of the battlefield or the 9/11 situation (Difede & Hoffman, 2002) using "computer graphics, body tracking devices, visual displays and other sensory input devices to immerse a participant in a computer-generated virtual environment that changes in a natural way with head and body motion" (Rothbaum, et al., 1999. p. 263).

THE COUNTING METHOD

Frank Ochberg's (1996) counting method is a simple therapy for a single event or simple trauma. The therapist directs the client to spend about 2 minutes silently imagining a specific event from beginning to end, while the therapist counts aloud from 1 to 100. The client gets to the worst or most intense part by 40s, 50s, and 60s and begins to wind down, finishing the event in the 90s. At 94, the therapist says, "Back here." After 100, the therapist waits for the client to open eyes, make contact, and talk about it. The therapist is supportive and affirming of the client's experience and the courage for going through the exercise. For a simple trauma, "three to five counting sessions are usually sufficient to help the client feel a sense of mastery and control over the intrusive recollections of that particular trauma. . . . [More complex trauma] may require a number of consecutive sessions or several sessions spaced months apart" (Johnson, Hadar, & Ochberg, 2007, p. 10).

Since clients don't speak during the counting, it allows them to have privacy while they recall their traumatic event. The exposure is time limited, 100 to 120 seconds, so that avoidant clients can be talked into doing it. It is exposure with a dual attention that can help clients stay oriented to the present while they imaginally move through their traumatic events.

Counting Method Resource

See the Counting Method Web site (http://www.countingmethod .com/) for information on the method, training, and its comprehensive handbook.

CLINICAL WRAP-UP

Exposure, bringing a client's attention to the traumatic event and the emotions tied to it, is a component of most trauma therapies. Many of the simple exposure therapies are easy to learn and easy to do. They cut to the chase of dealing with avoidance and creating trauma-based activation, two necessary components of healing PTSD. There are many venues for learning exposure therapies. Many graduate schools teach exposure as their favored trauma technique. Any larger city will host at least one exposure-based therapy training per year.

Exposure therapy on its own may retraumatize trauma survivors. It needs deep relational containment and careful titration or it can lead clients to drop out of therapy, self-medicate with alcohol or drugs, or become deeply hopeless, depressed, and suicidal. Many clients refuse to do EX. Classic EX is best with single-incident trauma, for it can overwhelm complex trauma clients who are not yet stabilized, leading to dissociative reactions, deep shame, and loss of control.

CHAPTER EIGHT

Cognitive Behavior Therapy

Cognitive behavior therapy (CBT), like exposure, is from the behavioral lineage. The idea is that if thoughts are behaviors, reinforced by classical and operant conditioning, then trauma survivors can learn to change their thoughts, thus changing their internal experience and external behaviors. CBT emphasizes the present over the past and deals with current self-defeating behaviors and thoughts. With its emphasis on the here and now, it dovetails nicely with mindfulness techniques. While many CBT therapies have an exposure component, some don't. This chapter presents a few of the many CBT therapies.

According to Marcia Herival (personal communication, October 27, 2009), "CBT is for people operating under cognitive distortions, because of what happened to them. All cognitive therapies deal with the triangle of thoughts, feelings, and actions. The point of CBT is to show the connection between the triangle points and how one point influences the others."

RATIONAL EMOTIVE BEHAVIOR THERAPY

Albert Ellis's rational emotive behavior therapy (REBT) was developed in the 1950s and is still in use. REBT follows the ABC model: Adversity or Activating event happens and contributes to the disturbance. Beliefs about the event contribute to the emotional and behavioral Consequences. By intervening with the Beliefs, you change the meaning of the Adverse event and thus change the emotional Consequences. In 1980, when I first read a transcript of an REBT session, it looked a lot like Ellis was arguing with the client. In fact, he was. Unlike the ISTDP practitioners, who push their clients into affective experience, Ellis argued about the meaning of events and thoughts relating to the client's self. He challenged self-defeating ideas like, "Now that this bad thing has occurred, I'm ruined for life" and, "I shouldn't be affected by this." One of his favorite targets was the belief, "I should have been perfect."

REBT teaches unconditional acceptance of self, others, and life; that we humans are fallible and imperfect and that we had better get used to it; and that we can't always get what we want, so we need to make the best of what we can and can't change. The goal is orderly mind, emotions, and actions. REBT therapists work as teachers and coaches, not necessarily warm and caring containers. They look at target problems, set goals, and assess affect, beliefs, especially core beliefs, and actions. First, the client acknowledges the problems, accepts emotional responsibility, and states motivation to change. Therapists coach the client to confront their self-abnegating and negative thoughts, affect, and actions. It can look like a debate or a Socratic dialogue. Therapists give homework, sometimes exposure or desensitization exercises in confronting feared tasks, people, or situations. Successful REBT clients accept themselves, their limitations, their situations, and the people around them.

REBT Resources for Therapists

Albert Ellis and Windy Dryden, *The Practice of Rational Emotive Behavior Therapy*, 2nd ed. (Springer, 2007).

Albert Ellis and Catharine MacLaren, *Rational Emotive Behavior Therapy: A Therapist's Guide*, 2nd ed. (Impact Publishers, 2005).

REBT Resources for Laypeople

Albert Ellis, *Feeling Better, Getting Better, Staying Better* (Impact Publishers, 2001).

Albert Ellis et al., *A Guide to Rational Living*, 3rd rev. ed. (Wilshire, 1997).

COGNITIVE THERAPY

Aaron Beck developed cognitive therapy (CT) to treat depression, then anxiety, then PTSD. CT targets distorted or unreasonably negative habitual "automatic thoughts," which influence affect, cognitive processing, and our bodily states. CT clients learn to identify, challenge, and evaluate these unhelpful cognitions, then replace them with more suitable, logical, or helpful thoughts. CT trauma clients work with ideas about their safety, "danger, trust, and views of themselves" (Rothbaum et al., 2000, p. 66). Schiraldi (2000, pp. 154–155) shows that Beck goes after catastrophizing thoughts: "These intrusions are unbearable." "It's awful to feel these bad feelings." Fortune-telling thoughts: "If I let myself feel, I'll lose control and never stop crying. I'll go crazy." "I'll never feel safe again." Personalizing thoughts: "It was my fault I was raped." Beck and other CT practitioners counter these thoughts and teach clients to counter them with antidotes: "The intrusion is okay. It's just a manifestation of my trauma." "These bad feelings are just a sign that I can still feel. Good feelings will return." "I can stand it even if I don't like it." And for thoughts of losing control or never feeling better: "Feelings don't make people go crazy. Crying always stops and is better than shutting down." "Life isn't safe, but if I take care, I might feel reasonably safe." "No one deserves to be raped. The cause was the perpetrator; not me. I'm not responsible for a crime, only my recovery."

CT antidotes are always logical and often what a therapist or anybody would say to a trauma survivor. Clients are taught to stop the negative thoughts and counter them with positive support thoughts in and out of the office. Beck and other clinicians use thought-stopping techniques, including having their clients shout "Stop!" while imagining a big red stop sign, to prevent breaking into repetitive distressing thoughts or intrusive images.

Beck mentored David Burns, the prolific writer of CT self-help books. They and other CT therapists have compiled lists of hundreds of cognitive distortions and how to counter them in workbooks, homework assignments, and CT training, all over the world.

CT Resources for Clinicians

Beck has published many books, and hundreds have been published overall. The following are a few of Beck's that have trauma components.

A. T. Beck, *Cognitive Therapy and the Emotional Disorders* (International Universities Press, 1975).

J. Scott, J. M. Williams, and A. T. Beck, *Cognitive Therapy in Clinical Practice: An Illustrative Casebook* (Routledge, 1989).

A. T. Beck, A. Freeman, and D. D. Davis, *Cognitive Therapy of Personality Disorders* (Guilford, 2003).

A. T. Beck, G. Emery, and R. L. Greenberg, *Anxiety Disorders and Phobias: A Cognitive Perspective* (Basic Books, 2005).

D. D. Burns, *Therapist's Toolkit: Comprehensive Treatment and Assessment Tools for the Mental Health Professional* (Philadelphia: Author, 1995; updated in 1997 and 2006).

D. R. Ledley, B. P. Marx, and R. G. Heimberg, *Making Cognitive-Behavioral Therapy Work: Clinical Process for New Practitioners* (Guilford, 2005).

CT Resources for Clients

Again, there are hundreds of books for clients. I list a few here.

D. D. Burns, *Feeling Good: The New Mood Therapy* (Revised and updated, Avon Books, 1999).

D. D. Burns, *When Panic Attacks* (Morgan Road Books, 2006).

G. R. Schiraldi, *The Post-Traumatic Stress Disorder Sourcebook* (Lowell House, 2000). Chapters 20–22 have step-by-step instructions for countering negative thoughts and emotions pertaining directly to trauma.

COGNITIVE PROCESSING THERAPY

Patricia Resick and Monica Schnicke (1992, 1993) developed cognitive processing therapy (CPT) to address the whole range of the emotions (including shame) in rape survivors with PTSD; the meaning of the elements of their traumatic memory; and to look at the accommodation that survivors made in their response to their sexual trauma. CPT therapists coach clients through filling out many worksheets including the Challenging Questions Worksheet, the Faulty Thinking Patterns Worksheet, and the Challenging Beliefs Worksheet. CPT is a highly structured therapy that follows the same path with each client. It involves daily homework, a strict focus on thoughts, and a very specific schedule. There may be a set number of sessions, often dealing with these topics:

1. Psychoeducation, an explanation of PTSD.

2. Exposure, remembering the traumatic event while identifying thoughts and feelings.

3. Impact statement about what the traumatic event means to the client and her beliefs about it. Therapists identify "stuck points" or cognitive distortions and find out if the trauma has changed beliefs about the self or the world.

4. Writing about the trauma, in session, focusing on sensory experience, emotions, beliefs, and thoughts. The client rereads it daily, at home.

5. The therapist teaches the client to question her distorted beliefs, sometimes using the Socratic method. "I don't understand. You were a little girl. How was it your fault that a big adult assaulted you? What could you have done about it?"

6. Identification of stuck points.

7. Going after faulty thinking patterns.

8. Working with trust and safety issues.

9. Power and control issues.

10. Esteem issues.

11. Intimacy issues (Shiperd, Street, & Resick, 2006).

There is a tremendous amount of homework, including filling out forms for each issue area and rereading the rewritten trauma narrative. CPT teaches clients to develop an internal Albert Ellis. It even employs Ellis's ABC model. One worksheet heading has three columns:

1. Activating Event: Something happens.

2. Beliefs: I tell myself something.

3. Consequence: I feel.

CPT Resources

Patty Resick and Monica Schnicke, *Cognitive Processing Therapy for Rape Victims: A Treatment Manual* (Sage, 1993).

DISCUSSION OF COGNITIVE THERAPIES

There are hundreds of books, trainings, homework resources, and audio CDs for cognitive therapists. These therapies have easy conceptual frameworks and logical step-by-step procedures, and are widely accepted by insurance companies. They can work well for cognitively oriented clients who have the wherewithal to access their left-brain cognitive functions to do homework and engage intellectually with their therapists. CBT can be used with other therapies that have more right brain and body focus.

Clients who are overwhelmed with emotions and flashbacks don't have their left brains online to do cognitive processing. Many of the simpler CBT therapies don't recognize the altered states and dissociation of complex PTSD. When overwhelmed with unmyelinated ventral vagal trauma states that shut down many left-brain functions, some CBT clients can feel like failures for being unable to feel good, to defeat PTSD symptoms, or to concentrate on the cognitive tasks of CT. For many years, I've been receiving clandestine referrals from a CBT-only agency, after clients failed there. These clients were able to completely clear their PTSD symptoms by more right-brain inclusive means. CBT therapies don't always eradicate trauma symptoms. Often they help people accept being traumatized. Other modalities may eradicate the symptoms, leaving clients trauma-free and automatically upgrading their negative cognitions to positive acceptance of self and a sense of safety in the world.

STRESS INOCULATION THERAPY

Stress inoculation therapy (SIT) helps people cope with stressful events after they happen and tries to inoculate them against future and ongoing stressors (Meichenbaum, 1996). Its goal is to help clients "gain confidence in their ability to cope with anxiety and fear stemming from reminders of their trauma" (Tull, 2009). In SIT's conceptualization phase, therapists or "trainers" use a Socratic-type dialogue to educate clients about stress and trauma and how thoughts and assessment might exacerbate their distress. Clients learn to see new stressors as problems to solve, and compare what they can do about problems with what they can't. They learn to cut big stressors into bite-size problems to be solved.

In the second phase, SIT clients acquire skills and rehearse what they learned in the first phases, first in the office, then out in the real world with their real problems. Specific skills include emotional self-regulation, self-soothing and acceptance, relaxation training, self-instructional training, cognitive restructuring, problem solving, communication skills training, attention diversion procedures, using social support systems, and fostering meaning-related activities.

In the third and last phase, application and follow-through, clients apply their coping skills with increasing levels of stressors. Therapists use imagery, imaginal rehearsal, role-playing, and modeling appropriate behavior. Clients may work with other clients to teach them the skills. Clients also learn relapse prevention, by anticipating ongoing or probable future triggers, and attribution, in which clients take credit for their changes.

SIT is used in a variety of settings, for individuals and groups, for past trauma or stress, or prophylactically, as a preparation for likely stressful or traumatic situations. It's used by the military, to prepare first-time combatants to deal with the stress of combat, for treatment of PTSD, and to prepare traumatized soldiers to return to battle.

SIT Resources

Donald Meichenbaum, *Stress Inoculation Training* (Allyn and Bacon, 1985).

Donald Meichenbaum, "Stress Inoculation Training for Coping With Stressors" (available at http://www.apa.org/divisions/div12/rev_est/sit_stress.html). A brief article with a good description.

ACCEPTANCE AND COMMITMENT THERAPY

According to Walser and Hayes, "Acceptance and Commitment Therapy (ACT) is a behaviorally based intervention designed to target and reduce experiential avoidance and cognitive entanglement while encouraging clients to make life-enhancing behavioral changes that are in accord with their personal values. . . . ACT helps clients make room for their difficult memories, feelings, and thoughts as they are directly experienced, and to include these experiences as part of a valued whole life" (2006, pp. 146–147). According to founder Stephen Hayes, ACT's goals are to induce a state of "creative hopelessness" in clients, so they realize that what they've been doing so far hasn't worked. They learn that their problem is trying to control, rather than accept the flashbacks and distressing emotions; understand that they are the context rather than the content of their emotions and thoughts; learn that they must let go of the agenda of maintaining control over thoughts, feelings, memories, or body sensations; and must make a commitment to their values and the new behaviors that arise from them (Hayes, Strosahl, & Wilson, 1999). Walser and Westrup articulate the goals that the therapist and client need to have together: "an awareness of what sort of life the client would ideally be living; recognition of what has stood in the way; awareness that most of the perceived barriers are not actual barriers; and awareness that one has [the] ability to make choices in the direction of that desired life" (2007, p. 40).

ACT is behavioral therapy that borrows or reinvents components of other good therapies:

- Mindfulness: ACT therapists teach that trauma-driven thoughts, sensations, and behaviors can be held in the larger context of mindful awareness. They coach clients through a variety of mindfulness exercises, so that they become observers of their internal processes, developing themselves as larger contexts for their internal experience. Mindfulness exercises can include body scans and classic meditation techniques of watching thoughts go by like leaves on the wind, walking meditation, and others.

- Acceptance: Clients learn to accept rather than avoid negative thoughts, sensations, their own fallibility, and their whole selves, through mindful awareness and cognitive therapy techniques. They learn to accept that the past is past and true, and to focus on and accept the present and move into the future.

- Exposure: ACT "specifically endeavors to expose clients to difficult emotional and thought experiences while promoting efforts to remain present rather than escaping the feared experiences . . . [though] ACT views avoidance as a more global strategy" than do strictly exposure therapies, which focus solely on traumatic events (Walser & Westrup, 2007, p. 207). ACT, like other cognitive therapies, addresses a range of negative thoughts about the self and the world. ACT is more about acceptance, "having what you have," and staying with whatever that internal experience and external reality is. Walser and Westrup find ACT to be a good lead-up or concurrent therapy to classic exposure therapy.

- Narrative: ACT strives to "deliteralize language and establish self as context" (Walser & Hayes, 2006, p. 164), including imagery exercises that are based in hypnotic practice such as turning thoughts and emotions into solid objects that can be examined; the meditative practice of watching thoughts float down the stream of awareness; and the exposure-based practice of repeating negative thoughts up to hundreds of times, until the client is desensitized. ACT also teaches helpful metaphors that give a context for expanded thinking and consciousness.

- Behavior changes: ACT clients identify their values and goals, then commit to new valued behaviors. They focus on what's doable, whatever their level of traumatization. And they explore, with their posttrauma identities, willingness and commitment to change and current and future vitality in life.

ACT Resources

Robyn Walser and Darrah Westrup, *Acceptance and Commitment Therapy for the Treatment of Post-Traumatic Stress Disorders and Trauma Related Problems* (New Harbinger Publications, 2007). A clear easy read, with great examples, that takes you step by step through the theory and practice of ACT for trauma. The book includes a CD with all the worksheets and exercises from the book.

Many trainings are available in the U.K. and Australia, with growing availability in the United States.

ACT Discussion

ACT is a comprehensive therapy that addresses the therapeutic relationship, acceptance of one's circumstances and one's self, mindfulness while experiencing trauma reactions, and commitment to new, value-supported action, whatever the current traumatic experience. Many ACT components can be integrated with other therapies to good avail. I use creative hopelessness and commitment to new behaviors with many clients.

Like most CBT-based therapies, ACT addresses dissociation tangentially, as avoidance. The ACT model assumes that people will learn to live with and accept their continuing PTSD symptoms. Other methods completely clear most trauma, so that clients don't have to accept lifelong distress. Use ACT methods with EMDR, thought field therapy, and ego state work to bring in mindfulness, acceptance, and commitment to future action, while completely clearing trauma symptoms.

DIALECTICAL BEHAVIOR THERAPY

See Chapter 21, "Treatments for Borderline Personality Disorder," for an examination of dialectical behavior therapy, a CBT and mindfulness treatment for complex trauma.

CHAPTER NINE

Eye Movement Desensitization and Reprocessing

Call it EMDR. Think of it as "reprocessing therapy." First, EMDR's "eye movements" are only one form of bilateral stimulation (BLS), which can be alternating hand taps, hand pulsers, or headsets playing alternating tones or music. "Desensitization" isn't right either. Think of associative and integrative therapy. Desensitization is exposure to something until your brain gives up responding to it. EMDR connects the "here and now" parts of your brain to the "there and then" trauma parts, until your brain says, "Oh, it's over. I'm okay." If EMDR's developer, Francine Shapiro, knew 20 years ago what she knows now, she'd call it reprocessing therapy. However, it's called EMDR and we'll stick with that.

EMDR is a therapy for the entire spectrum of trauma. With well-attached, affect-tolerant clients, you can often completely clear one-event traumas in a few sessions. What does clearing mean? It means that clients can hold a traumatic event in mind while experiencing no symptoms of PTSD: no negative cognitions, no old, bad sensations, no flashbacks, and later, no bad dreams. Of course, the more pervasive the trauma—years in a war zone or a horrific childhood—the more sessions you need. You can use EMDR to transform the "small t" (F. Shapiro, 2001) relational traumas and attachment deficits that create so many personality, attachment, and secondary dissociation disorders. And tied with ego state therapies, you can use it to clear the catastrophic attachment and pervasive trauma of tertiary dissociation: DID and DDNOS (Forgash & Copeley, 2008; Paulsen, 2009).

One of the simplest ways of describing EMDR effects is to say that the target event has remained unprocessed because the immediate biochemical responses to the trauma have left it isolated in neurobiological stasis. When the client tracks a moving finger or attends to hand taps, tones, or even a fixed point on a wall, active information processing is initiated to attend to the present stimulus. If the client is asked to attend simultaneously both to this stimulus and to the traumatic memory, the active information-processing mechanism is linked to and processes the target event as well as the current stimulus. This processing mechanism is physiologically configured to take the information to an adaptive resolution. (F. Shapiro, 2001, p. 323)

EMDR includes elements of mindfulness, somatic awareness, exposure, and cognitive therapies. See if you spot them all in the eight phases that follow.

THE EIGHT PHASES OF EMDR

EMDR is an eight-phase approach with protocols that attend to three prongs: past events that set the foundation for pathology, current situations that cause disturbance, and future templates for appropriate future action. Francine Shapiro's (2001) amended standard protocol follows.

- Phase 1, client history, includes client readiness, client safety factors, and dissociation screening. Targets are identified to address past, present, and future. Safety, readiness, and dissociation assessment are mandatory. Many of us say the fastest way to find undiagnosed DID is to do EMDR without screening.
- Phase 2, preparation, includes creating a bond with the client, setting expectations, creating a safe place, and testing the eye movements or other BLS. This can happen in one session with a one-occurrence trauma or take months with someone with terrible attachment and nonexistent affect regulation.
- Phase 3, assessment, is the beginning of trauma processing and includes selecting the picture that represents the target, identifying the negative cognition, developing a positive cognition, rating the validity of cognition, naming the emotion, estimating the subjective units of disturbance, and identifying body sensa-

tions. The brilliant beginning of trauma processing brings together the image, cognitions, emotions, and body sensations. Daniel Siegel (2003), when asked why EMDR works, said that the bilateral stimulation begins in phase 3, by starting with the image and hopping from left-brain cognitions to right-brain emotions to left-brain measuring while holding the emotion, to right-brain body-mapping.

- Phase 4, desensitization, includes reprocessing the memory using BLS in sets of varying length, depending on the client's response, until the trauma is completely cleared. Eye movements are most often used and may be the most effective. BLS seems to stimulate the integrative capacity of the brain. Some think that the dual attention—clients remembering and feeling while paying attention to the here-and-now BLS—is part of why it works. Others think that the bilaterality stimulates the connection across the corpus callosum. Robert Stickgold (2001), a sleep researcher, thinks that BLS stimulates a REM-like state that helps process the undigested trauma.

- Phase 5 is installing the positive cognition. While holding the memory in mind, the client is able to completely endorse the positive cognition; for example, "It's over." "I'm safe now." "I'm blameless." "I'm lovable." At this point, the client no longer feels the trauma inside and usually can endorse the original positive cognition while thinking of the traumatic event.

- Phase 6, body scan, is searching for any bodily disturbance and continuing to process until it's completely gone. "Go through your whole body, noticing any distressing sensation. Focus on that, and we'll do more eye movements."

- Phase 7, closure, includes homework to monitor changes, expectations, and, if needed, bringing the client to a state of emotional equilibrium. Clients who are working on huge or repeated trauma may need to be brought back to their safe places or use containers to get back to themselves. If the trauma isn't completely cleared, flashbacks of old or even newer material may pop up between sessions.

- Phase 8, reevaluation, includes checking in at the next session to see if the client requires new processing for the previous target or associated material. Because EMDR wakes up material that's associated with the original trauma, your client may come to the next session with a new, but related, target.

TYPICAL SESSION

As a client in a typical EMDR processing session, you reconnect with your therapist, check in on last week's work, and pick your processing target. Your therapist reminds you about your safe place and that you get a break from processing anytime you need one. You imagine the worst part of the traumatic event, say what outdated thought comes with it ("I'm not safe. I'm bad."), what you'd rather think ("It's over. I'm safe. I'm blameless."), and how true that positive cognition feels. You say what emotion goes with it, measure that emotion and where you feel it, and immediately start the BLS. Then the therapist gets out of the way and lets your brain direct the work. He or she monitors you closely until you shift, sigh, nod, or otherwise show that that set is done. You reconnect with your therapist between each set, say briefly what you notice, then go back to the BLS. Usually the trauma becomes more intense. You start to remember more and more, and the processing often goes forward in time through the whole event. If either the event or those kinds of feelings connect to other times, those situations start to come up in your mind. You might start with the latest car accident and then remember the other three accidents and the time you almost drowned. Then all of the feelings tied to those events start to fade. After a number of sets of BLS, your therapist asks you to think of the original event. If there's still more "juice" in the event, you do more processing until the trauma is gone. When it's finally gone, your body doesn't have the sensations or the emotions, and it's easy to believe that it's over, you're safe, and it wasn't your fault that the drunk driver rammed into you. You think of the accident and say, "I'm safe," and it feels true. You scan your body, and it feels warm and light. When you think of the accident, you can still remember it, but it's off in the distance, just a memory, and it doesn't bother you again.

EMDR TARGETS

You can use the standard protocol on a variety of targets including distressing physical sensations, eating disorders, phantom and chronic pain (Wilson & Tinker, 2005), beliefs about the self (Knipe, 2005), anxiety disorders, and depression (Manfield, 1998). I've written about using EMDR to clear familial and cultural introjects, traumatic couples issues, anxiety disorders, some forms of depression, obsessive-compulsive personality disorder, medical trauma, and multiple chemical sensitivities (R. Shapiro, 2005, 2009a, 2009b). The EMDR clinical literature tends to tell you how and on what targets and in what order you should focus the standard protocol. Remember the strategic developmental model from Chapter 3? That was developed to create an efficient way to process targets in complex cases.

Children are the best subjects for EMDR. They process more quickly than adults. In the time an adult would be just getting started, a child will say "Done" and mean it. Some modify the protocol for smaller children. I modify it for adolescents. If they don't want to tell me exactly what we're targeting, I don't make them. Sometimes, we do the setup and the clearing, the distress goes away, and they may or may not tell me about it later. Some boys like it because they don't have to talk too much when in therapy. Boys often like the technology (pulsers and flashing lights) that go with the way I do EMDR. Several clinicians have found ways to use stories with embedded EMDR to work with children (Greenwald, 1999; Lovett, 1999; Turner, 2005).

COMPLEX TREATMENT FOR COMPLEX CASES

Sometimes the standard protocol is not enough. EMDR clinicians use ego state therapy (Forgash & Copeley, 2008; Paulsen, 2009; Paulsen & Lanius, 2009), dialectical behavior therapy techniques (Lovell, 2005), somatic therapies (Paulsen & Lanius, 2009), hypnotherapy, and techniques from many other kinds of therapy to stabilize, connect with, and contain highly reactive or dissociative clients. Sometimes, therapists alter the standard protocol, such as leaving out attention to bodily sensation in highly abreactive clients. Other times they add pieces in, shorten processing sets, or target very small, specific pieces of trauma. Good EMDR therapists take time to prepare their fragile and highly dissociative clients with resource installation (Leeds, 2009; Kiessling, 2005), calming techniques, and a good solid therapeutic relationship before embarking on trauma processing, and may go back to resourcing and calming at the end of processing to increase stabilization between sessions.

CAVEATS

Why do clinicians take so much care with fragile EMDR clients? Because this powerful technique often takes minutes to break through decades of emotional defense and dissociation. If you want your most distressed clients to stay alive, intact, and in therapy, you will help them titrate the reexperiencing of affect and cognitions that went with years of horrible abuse. To do that you have to have tools in place and enough therapeutic relationship to call your client out of the morass, or to enter the morass slowly and in control. Don't try to do EMDR without formal training. It's so powerful you can hurt people with it, if you don't know what you're doing.

SUMMARY

EMDR is a powerful associative and integrative technique that uses visual, cognitive, and sensory cues to concentrate a trauma and then BLS alternating with connection to the therapist to clear traumas across the trauma spectrum. When it works, and it most often does, it makes trauma symptoms disappear.

RESOURCES

Training

- EMDR Humanitarian Assistance Program: EMDR-HAP provides inexpensive and, if they have a grant, free training to therapists in nonprofit agencies, the military and Veteran's Administration, and underserved communities in the United States and around the world. They also support a volunteer network that responds to local and faraway disasters. Contact them at http://www.emdrhap.org, if you want to explore bringing a training to your nonprofit or to support their cause.
- EMDR Institute: Francine Shapiro's training organization (http://www.emdr.com).

- To find an independent EMDR trainer, go to http://www .emdria.org and find Basic EMDR Training Sites.

Books

The following are a few of the 29 EMDR-related books published, as of 2009.

For Laypeople

Francine Shapiro and Margot Silk Forrest, *EMDR: The Breakthrough Therapy for Overcoming Anxiety, Stress, and Trauma* (Basic Books, 1997).

Laurel Parnell, *Transforming Trauma: EMDR* (Norton, 1997).

Barb Maiberger, *EMDR Essentials: A Guide for Clients and Therapists* (Norton, 2009).

The Basics

Francine Shapiro, *Eye Movement Desensitization and Reprocessing: Basic Principles, Protocols, and Procedures* (Guilford, 2001). The bible of EMDR.

Laurel Parnell, *A Therapist's Guide to EMDR: Tools and Techniques for Successful Treatment* (Norton, 2007). More accessible than the "bible."

Andrew Leeds, *A Guide to the Standard EMDR Protocols for Clinicians, Supervisors, and Consultants* (Springer, 2009).

EMDR With Children

Ana Gomez, *Dark, Bad Day . . . Go Away!* (2007). A lovely children's storybook that's an introduction to EMDR. Available from http://www.emdrhap.org

Robbie-Adler Tapia and Carolyn Settle, *EMDR and the Art of Psychotherapy With Children* (Springer, 2008).

Ricky Greenwald, *EMDR in Child and Adolescent Psychotherapy* (Jason Aronson, 1999).

Joan Lovett, *Small Wonders: Healing Childhood Trauma With EMDR* (Simon and Schuster, 1999).

Robert Tinker and Sandra Wilson, *Through the Eyes of a Child: EMDR With Children* (Norton, 1999).

Special Populations

Steven M. Silver and Susan Rogers, *Light in the Heart of Darkness: EMDR and the Treatment of War and Terrorism Survivors* (Norton, 2002).

Carol Forgash and Margaret Copeley (Eds.), *Healing the Heart of Trauma and Dissociation With EMDR and Ego State Therapy* (Springer, 2008). Wonderful chapters about ego states, neurobiology, and therapy in general.

Sandra Paulsen, *Looking Through the Eyes of Trauma and Dissociation: An Illustrated Guide for EMDR Therapists and Clients* (Bainbridge Institute for Integrative Psychology, 2009).

Philip Manfield (Ed.), *EMDR Casebook* (Norton, 2003). A step-by-step walk through treatment of depression, masochism, rage, guilt, war trauma, secondary traumatization, phobia, childhood abuse, shame, and narcissism.

Robin Shapiro (Ed.), *EMDR Solutions: Pathways to Healing* (Norton, 2005). The strategic development model, resource development, DID, opioid antagonists with DID, addiction, procrastination, cultural introjects, EMDR with dialectical behavior therapy, couples, binge-purge cycle, mentally disabled clients, anxiety disorders, and affect regulation with kids.

Robin Shapiro (Ed.), *EMDR Solutions II: For Depression, Eating Disorders, Performance, and More* (Norton, 2009). Contains chapters on working with depression, performance, coaching, EMDR prep, early trauma, EMDR with somatic and ego state interventions, complex trauma, obsessive-compulsive personality disorder, medical trauma, multiple chemical sensitivities, sex offenders, and religious issues. Includes seven chapters on eating disorders.

CHAPTER TEN

Somatic Therapies

As you remember the beating, bring your attention to your body. . . . What sensations are you noticing? . . . Your shoulders are tight? Can you exaggerate that tightness? That's right, pay attention to the sensation. What's happening with your arms? . . . Right, they look clamped down to your sides. Notice the sensations in your arms and shoulders. Is there a movement that your arms want to do? Slowly, slowly, paying attention to the feeling in your arms, let them start that movement. (Client slowly brings both hands in front of face in a defensive posture.)

What do they want to do now? Push? Before you start the pushing motion, could you sink into your legs? That's right. Bend your knees, feel the ground supporting you. How does that feel? More grounded? Great. Start that pushing motion, slowly, paying attention to the sensation in your arms. What's that like? "Scary, but strong." Keep going. Notice how your shoulders have dropped to support the pushing.

Keep noticing. Let yourself complete that movement, pushing all the way through from your shoulders to the ends of your hands. What's that like? "Strong and grounded." When you think of the beating, what do you notice, now? "More grounded and stronger, and I'm feeling more sensation in my legs."

Focus into your legs. . . . Stay with the sensations. . . . What do your legs want to do? Kick behind you? Sink into your legs so you can keep your balance. When you're ready, kick. Slow it down so your brain can process it. Great! Does the other foot need to kick? Go for it, paying attention to the feeling.

What do you notice now? "I want to kick from on the ground." Lie down on the mat and go for it, with full attention. Follow through all the way. And what are you noticing now? Another sensation? Itchy, prickly in your legs. Stay with it until it's done. . . . "I want to run away now." Go for it. Try slow motion so your brain can get it. . . .

What do you notice now when you think of the beating? "Relief. It feels over now. And relaxation." Do a scan through your whole body. What else do you get? "I feel strong, and alert, and I can't find any fear, now. I feel confident." Great! Where do you feel all that good stuff? And what movements does your body want to do while you're feeling strong, alert, fearless, and confident? Go for it!

There are many kinds of movement and somatic therapies. Most share the concept that trauma dysregulates the body, causing restrictions in emotions and movement; that unfinished movements from the time of the trauma need to be experienced; and that attention to sensation and movement will release the trauma, bringing the client's body and brain to a new equilibrium. Most somatic and movement therapies have elements of exposure (remembering the trauma) and mindfulness (noticing present-time experience). Some involve actual movement in the here and now, most often completing the held back, repressed, or "undone" movement from the traumatic event. Some involve attention to bodily sensations with little or no movement.

From the 1960s through the early 1990s, many movement therapies taught that catharsis was the way to move through old traumas. Clients would punch pillows or the air, kick, sob, scream, and writhe on the floor. After these therapies many people, especially those with simple PTSD, found that they had more affect tolerance and more freedom of movement and expression, felt more relaxed and more powerful, and were no longer plagued by PTSD symptoms. Clients with deeper trauma and higher levels of dissociation were often left unhealed or even damaged by these therapies. Some would express their trauma while in a single dissociative state (i.e., a "fight" emotional part) without integrating their experience, having the same experience over and over with temporary state changes, but no long-term change of symptoms. Others would decompensate to the point of hospitalization or be triggered to act out old scenarios on unsuspecting movement therapy group members or staff.

Newer somatic therapies move more slowly, tracking clients closely as they track their own process. They often include relational or emotional holding by the therapist and have less emphasis on catharsis and more on rebalancing the nervous system through slow attention to sensation and affect.

SOMATIC EXPERIENCING

Peter Levine, a physiologist and psychologist, uses somatic experiencing (SE) to focus on the physical effects of trauma. In his 1997 book, *Waking the Tiger*, he emphasizes the freeze response, noting that most animals are programmed to reorient and calm down after trauma and that humans, with our big, complex brains, need conscious awareness to bring on our orienting response and the physical, emotional, and mental homeostasis in which we function best. Referring to Porges's polyvagal theory from Chapter 2, Levine helps his clients to go from dorsal or shutdown states and sympathetic fight-flight states to ventral vagal, interested, connectable states.

Levine notes that when animals go from a hypervigilant state to a normal relaxed activity state, "they often begin to vibrate, twitch, and lightly tremble. . . . These little tremblings of muscular tissue are the organism's way of regulating extremely different states of nervous system activation" (1997, pp. 97–98). For humans, "The fear of experiencing terror, rage, and violence toward oneself or others, or of being overwhelmed by the energy discharged in the mobilization process, keeps the human immobility response in place" (p. 104). He sees PTSD as cumulative, taking months or more for the freezing response to become chronic. He differentiates between "shock" or single-incident trauma that may be treated solely with SE in a few sessions and developmental trauma, which may take much longer and involve other kinds of therapy.

SE uses "pendulation," having clients shift focus between positive innate orienting responses and the freeze response, or active defensive bodily states. Clients are coached to stay with the subsequent shaking and release of pent-up energy, then directed to notice the next bodily area of tension and holding. Clients might imagine running away or fighting back, while noting the body's response to their imaginal actions. Therapists continue the process until the tension and trauma reactions dissipate and the client is in a relaxed and energized state of equilibrium.

SE is helpful for trauma but lacks the attachment components necessary for work with many complex trauma clients. Its techniques work well in combination with attachment-oriented therapies, in the context of a good containing therapeutic relationship.

SENSORIMOTOR PSYCHOTHERAPY

Sensorimotor psychotherapy (SP), developed and evolving since the 1980s by Pat Ogden, is a "body-oriented talking therapy" that intentionally integrates psychotherapy and body therapy (Ogden et al., 2006). SP helps clients stabilize, release, and heal the physiological symptoms of trauma, attachment failure, grief and loss, and developmental arrest by using a wide range of somatic interventions woven seamlessly into the psychotherapeutic process. SP emphasizes the need of the client to maintain a neurophysiological window of tolerance between hyper- and hypoarousal of the nervous system, in order for verbal interventions to be effective. SP is intentional in its differential use of "top-down" (cognition initiated) and "bottom-up" (sensory initiated) interventions to help the client maintain and expand that window. Also stressed is the role of physical movement, stillness, or collapse in symptom formation, and therapeutic use of physical movement and stillness in the healing process.

SP uses a three-phase treatment approach:

1. Development of somatic resources for stabilization

2. Trauma processing

3. Integration and success in normal life

In phase 1 the therapist assesses the client's physical being through microtracking and body reading, teaching the client to differentiate between emotion and sensation, to develop descriptive language for various sensations, to recognize bodily sensations when they are fragments of trauma memory, and to learn how and when to act, or not act, upon the felt sensations.

Phase 2 involves processing trauma and its effects. If the client's emotional and physiological arousal level begins to move outside the window of tolerance, the therapist may instruct the client to "drop the content" or "drop the emotion" and stay in the here and now of the body sensation, following it through toward completion of action that may have been truncated at the time of the trauma. Processing is slow, deliberate, and likely to proceed in micromovements as body sensations lead the way to more positive cognitions and a sense of the event being in the past.

In phase 3, the client addresses issues that arise in the absence of direct trauma symptoms, such as relationships and intimacy, vocation, and daily life. "Again, the therapist and clients track and study the emergent micromovements of the body, attending particularly to core versus peripheral body movement, with positive shifts in cognition and affect arising out of the work" (Martha Jacobi, 2009, unpublished manuscript).

Somatic Transformation

Sharon Stanley teaches somatic transformation, which includes interpersonal neurobiology (Schore, 1994, 2009; Porges, 2001, 2005), attachment throughout the life cycle, dissociative disorders, and somatic therapy within a relational model of therapy. She integrates somatic processes into depth psychology and teaches a rich, somatically based, psychotherapy-informed way of working.

Somatic Work With a Dissociative Client

He was in his early 40s, DDNOS, a survivor of catastrophic early neglect and abuse at the hands of his psychopathic father. After years of therapy, including ego state work and EMDR in the context of attachment therapy, the unfinished defensive movements began to arise throughout his body. His hands would spontaneously raise up, and his neck would spastically jerk to the left, over and over, in any context. His out-of-control body brought him deeper into shame, as it was, to him, another sign of his brokenness. As we slowly tracked the sensations in his neck and his arms, it became clear that the movements were in response to the hits he had taken to his head. For several sessions, and between sessions, he slowed the movement down, paid attention to the sensations and emotions that arose, and slowly completed the movement of turning away from the blows. If he'd turned away as a child, he would have been attacked more horribly. As he brought attention to his body, he was able to have compassion for the abused child he had been, and the shame began to dissipate. We were able to do some ego state work with the child state, coming to more integration, and the reflexive head turning dissipated.

Every day of his life, the client reexperienced physical sensations of the abuse, including the molestations and being hit. If we tried other kinds of trauma processing, he became flooded with the over-whelming sensations, cognitions, and emotions (fear and shame) of the time. Over and over, we used sensorimotor processing, focusing directly on the sensation until it slowly dissipated. Sometimes he would shake and twitch as the old muscular holding released. Sometimes his affect would change from shame to anger and an awareness of the unfairness of the abuse. At this writing, he still experiences old sensations, but not as pervasively, and with less distress.

RESOURCES

Somatic Experiencing

Peter Levine, *Waking the Tiger, Healing Trauma* (North Atlantic, 1997). This is the first book of the new wave of somatic therapies. He's written a do-it-yourself book that includes a CD with SE exercises, *Healing Trauma* (Sounds True, 2005).
Web site: http://www.traumahealing.com

Sensorimotor Psychotherapy

Pat Ogden, Kekuni Minton, and Clare Pain, *Trauma and the Body: A Sensorimotor Approach to Psychotherapy* (Norton, 2006). A deep good book about bodies, attachment, somatic work, and good therapy.
Web site: http://www.sensorimotorpsychotherapy.org/

Somatic Transformation

Web site: http://www.somatic-transformation.org

CHAPTER ELEVEN

Hypnotherapy

Clinical hypnosis creates state changes and sometimes creates permanent symptom eradication in traumatized people. Hypnotic techniques pervade many therapies. Hypnotherapists see their modality in guided imagery, ego state work, progressive relaxation, and the sing-song soothing tones used by many therapists. Some see dissociation, including PTSD, as a form of involuntary self-hypnosis. They "fight fire with fire" and use voluntary inductions to transform trauma symptoms (Calof, personal communication, September 3, 2009). With hypnosis you can enhance rapport, relaxation, introspection, and awareness and tolerance for sensations and emotions. You can shift your clients' trauma symptoms from the front burner to the back burner and then completely out of the kitchen.

TRANCE INDUCTIONS

As you sit in your comfortable chair reading this book, feeling the weight of the book in your hands and the weight of your body in the chair, you may already be wondering if you are in a light trance, and wondering how you know that, and noticing how your body might tell you that you know what you know and you can know that you already know that you can learn that there are hundreds of trance inductions that I don't have room to teach you, and that you can, when you're ready, see some of the many books and resources about them at the end of the chapter. (That's one induction.)

Inductions are simply ways to help clients become more focused in their attention. They can be as simple as, "Go inside, and find the answer to that question." Or they may involve elaborate ways of showing clients that they're in trance. Formal trance inductions include everything from "you're getting sleepy" to hand levitations and other structured hierarchies of deepening trance. Informal hypnosis may involve constant use of suggestive language ("As you sit on the chair and your eyes close, you might be wondering how deep you can go. And as you notice gravity holding you in that chair and your breath going in and out, you might find that you are going even deeper"), confusion and distraction techniques, storytelling, metaphors, or asking a client to talk to a particular age or part of self.

Good hypnotherapists closely follow clients' responses, collaborating with both the conscious and unconscious minds.

TREATING TRAUMA

David Calof, the Northwest's top hypnotherapist and a disciple of Milton Erickson, the famously innovative hypnotherapist, says that since traumatized and dissociative people naturally use trance, you often don't need to do formal inductions with them. Hypnosis can give them an internal locus of control and quick symptom relief, which builds confidence that change is possible, and a commitment to stay in therapy to go after all of the trauma symptoms. He uses hypnotherapy to teach preparation skills: relaxation, safe places, respite or sanctuary from internal and external stresses, presence, mindfulness, and openness to internal process. He does parts work (see Chapter 19) to identify and grow compassion among parts. He aids clients to build ego strength and address self-injury and substance abuse.

Specific Trauma Techniques of David Calof

These are the bare bones of examples of trauma techniques. They don't include all of the many words, inflections, and pauses that make a successful hypnotic intervention.

Detriggering or Symptom Recueing

"Whenever a flashback begins, the more you'll relax inside."

Distancing Techniques

1. A library of memories from which you can check out whatever we'll work on today (see container exercise at the end Chapter 4 for a full example).

2. A movie of the event. This can be used with material that is held by one part and denied by another. Describe the situation in the third person: "There was a little girl with dark hair who [describe someone like the client and whatever happened to the client]. Whenever it is okay with you, it will slowly dawn on you who that child is. And you will be able to deal with those feelings, now."

3. Affect dial to turn down or off the affect associated with trauma. I use TV remotes. "When I say 'three,' you'll be able to turn the switch up and down." (Good for PTSD. Especially great for borderline personalities and DID.)

4. Selective attention (which is trance): "You can use your searchlight to spotlight what you want to see. What you spotlight is what you'll notice. One thing at a time. You can choose a wide beam to see more or a narrow beam to see just one thing for just one moment. And if that's too intense, you can spotlight something easy to see in a good time."

5. Looking back at the present time from a year, 5 years, or 20 years from now to see what you did that worked to solve the problem or to gain perspective.

6. See the safe place exercise at the end of Chapter 4.

Other Hypnotic Trauma Techniques

1. Key word: "Pick a word that goes with that situation in which you overcame [something the client overcame]. Imagine approaching this new situation with your key word. That's right. What happens? Now put it all behind you and count to 20."

2. Forgetting: "You don't need to remember. . . . When you approach that intersection it will be as if you'd never seen it before and you'll be curious about what it looks like and how it is to be there."

3. Tool kits. Give clients all the hypnotic and other tools you have (all hypnosis is self-hypnosis) and then let them know that they don't have to consciously remember to use the tools: "Your body knows better than you do and it will find a way to use these tools. . . . You have no idea what you'll find or what will happen, and what you do find might surprise you." Calof says that he's seen people have tremendous insights and breakthroughs between sessions when he left them with this one.

4. Healed future: Asking when will the client be healed and how did she get to healing.

5. Transforming sensory experience: "Where do you feel that sensation or pain in your body? How big is it? What color is it? What shape is it? What texture? What color would you like it to be? Change it. Shape? Size? Texture? What do you notice now that you've changed it? How do you want to transform it, now? Go for it! I wonder what you will do to completely change the way it is and the way it affects you?" (See the techniques called "bringing in the light" and "targeted light stream" from Chapter 4.)

6. Ego state work arose from hypnotherapy (see Chapter 19).

CLINICAL WRAP-UP

Hypnotherapy, on its own, can be a powerful trauma therapy. Any other modality you use can be enhanced with hypnotic awareness and techniques. Not all hypnotherapies are alike. Formulaic one-size-fits-all scripts don't necessarily fit all. Learn the theory, learn techniques, and experience hypnosis yourself in the process to be best able to let it take you where you don't yet know it can take you. You might already be wondering where that is and what it might be like to know how to use the language and skills of this technique.

RESOURCES

Books

Milton Erickson, with Ernest Rossi and Sheila Rossi, *Hypnotic Realities: The Induction of Clinical Hypnosis and Forms of Indirect Sug-*

gestion (Irvington, 1976). A classic from the godfather of hypnotherapy. Available used all over the Internet.

Jay Haley, *Uncommon Therapy: The Psychiatric Techniques of Milton H. Erickson, M.D.* (Norton, 1973, 1993). A look at Erickson through communication theory and strategic therapy lenses.

Stephen G. Gilligan, *Therapeutic Trances: The Cooperation Principle in Ericksonian Hypnotherapy* (Brunner/Mazel, 1987). From one of the best teachers around.

D. Corydon Hammond (Ed.), *Handbook of Hypnotic Suggestions and Metaphors* (American Society of Clinical Hypnosis, 1990).

Richard Bandler and John Grinder, *The Structure of Magic: A Book About Language and Therapy* (Science and Behavior Books, 1975); *The Structure of Magic II: A Book About Communication and Change* (Science and Behavior Books, 1975). Bandler and Grinder filmed the best therapists of the early 1970s and deconstructed exactly what they did, systemized what they found, and wrote books about it. Erickson was their biggest subject. Valuable books for any therapist.

David Calof, *The Couple Who Became Each Other and Other Tales of Healing From a Hypnotherapist's Casebook* (Bantam, 1996). A fascinating read.

Training

There are hypnosis training sessions all over the world. Not all of them are trauma centered. Find out which might be appropriate for trauma reduction. Watch out for cookie-cutter or nonprofessional training.

Stephen Gilligan's Trance Camp is a famous place to learn and experience clinical hypnosis. It's educational, transformational, and fun. He has other trainings throughout the year, not all about hypnotherapy (see http://www.stephengilligan.com/TRANCEcamp.html).

The American Society of Clinical Hypnosis sponsors regional workshops and, once you join, is a good resource for all things hypnotic. Check out their Web site (http://www.asch.net/regionalworkshops .htm).

CHAPTER TWELVE

Energy Psychology

Energy psychologies combine Western psychotherapy techniques with components of traditional Asian medical practices of acupuncture and meridian therapies. David Feinstein explains that energy psychologies

> combine physical interventions for regulating electrical signals or energy fields with mental involvement in a feeling, cognition, or behavior that is a target for change [exposure]. This simultaneous pairing of the physical activity and mental activation is believed to therapeutically alter the targeted response. . . . In energy psychology, as with other exposure-based treatments, exposure is achieved by eliciting . . . hyperarousal associated with a traumatic memory. . . . Unique to energy psychology is that extinction of this association is facilitated by 1) the manual stimulation of acupuncture and related points that are believed to 2) send signals to the amygdala and other brain structures that 3) quickly reduce hyperarousal. When the brain then reconsolidates the traumatic memory, the new association (to reduced hyperarousal or no hyperarousal) is retained. (2008, p. 199)

The therapies vary, though most include focusing on a thought, emotion, or negative event while tapping or rubbing acupuncture points or meridians. Psychotherapists may use energy psychology techniques alone or in combination with other therapies.

Acupuncture

Though it's not a psychotherapy, acupuncture treats the effects of PTSD by using needles and herbs to balance the energy flow of the body. If people are hyperaroused, acupuncture brings them down to earth. When people are depressed, acupuncture stimulates the chi in specific meridians to bring them up to normal function. Clients report feeling more clear-headed, less anxious, less depressed, and more balanced. Hollifield, Sinclair-Lian, Warner, and Hammerschlag (2007) found treatment effects at the same level as group cognitive behavior therapy. The treatment effects maintained for at least 3 months after the end of treatment. Some acupuncturists are using ear acupuncture with trauma survivors and report that clients sleep better, have fewer flashbacks, and are more balanced, neither hyperaroused nor hypoaroused.

I've found acupuncture to be a good adjunct to psychotherapy. It rouses the chronically depressed, calms down the anxious, and helps to rebalance distressed nervous systems. Clients who are loath to consider medications may be happy to go to regular acupuncture sessions. Find an acupuncturist with a calm manner and the ability to connect, who can give your clients another emotionally containing relationship.

Thought-Field Therapy

Thought-field therapy (TFT), developed by Roger Callahan, uses a series of step-by-step "algorithms" (Callahan & Trubo, 2002) that combine tapping sequences, neurolinguistic programming exercises, and exposure and cognitive-behavioral affirmations to alleviate trauma, phobias, and anxiety. TFT therapists use applied kinesiology (see http://www.appliedkinesiology.com/), also known as muscle testing, and a series of set questions to decide which tapping sequence to use. They check for "reversals" in the energy flow. Then they direct clients to tap on specific meridian points in a specific pattern. The center of each sequence is the Nine-Gamut, during which clients open and shut and roll their eyes, count, and hum, while tapping on the "gamut spot" (Triple Warmer point, to acupuncturists). TFT can make phobias, single-event PTSD, and distressing affects disappear nearly instantaneously and often permanently.

Roger Callahan, a clinical psychologist, has created a powerful technique. He has also garnered ill will in some of the therapy community by his high-pressure marketing tactics to both lay people and therapists, lawsuits against other practitioners, and expensive training. Yet many therapists use TFT to help manage affect in clients who can't stay in the room with their distress, to clear many phobias and PTSD, and to give clients a safe technique to calm symptoms between sessions.

Simple Trauma Session With TFT

When you think about the worst part of the accident, what do you notice? How distressing is that, from 1 to 10? It's a 9, okay. Let's go. Think about the accident and feel the distress. Now tap on the spots on the inside of your eyebrows. Ten times. That's right. Now those collarbone spots, ten times, now keep tapping the gamut spot on your hand. Close your eyes, open them, look down to the right, then the left, circle your eyes to the right, then the left. Now hum a tune for 5 seconds. Now count to five, and hum again. Now think about that accident again, and tap those eyebrow points. Good, now the collarbone points. Ten times. Now the back of your hand again, looking up, taking a deep breath, and letting your eyes come down. How distressed are you now when you think of that accident? A 2? Great! Let's do another round.

TFT Resources

Roger Callahan and Richard Trubo, *Tapping the Healer Within: Using Thought-Field Therapy to Instantly Conquer Your Fears, Anxieties, and Emotional Distress* (McGraw-Hill, 2002).

Web site: http://www.rogercallahan.com includes many training sites and dates.

EMOTIONAL FREEDOM TECHNIQUE

EFT treats the same issues as TFT, in a simpler way. Instead of having to find a particular algorithm, clients use one longer tapping sequence for most targets. Each iteration of the EFT protocol may take longer than a TFT algorithm, but since clients have to learn just one protocol, it's easier. Gary Craig, the founder of EFT, democratically gives away his basic protocol on his Web site and in his books.

Therapists who have learned both TFT and EFT say that there is very little difference between them.

EFT Resources

Gary Craig, *The EFT Manual* (Energy Psychology Press, 2008).
Gary Craig, *EFT for PTSD* (Energy Psychology Press, 2009).
Helena Fone, *Emotional Freedom Technique for Dummies* (For Dummies, 2008).
Web site: http://www.emofree.com, where you can download the protocol, free.

TAPAS ACUPRESSURE TECHNIQUE (TAT)

Tapas Fleming, an acupuncturist, created TAT for use with trauma and other emotional issues as an outgrowth of her work with people suffering from allergies. She has clients stimulate three points on their heads while reciting a series of positive affirmations. TAT has more of an obvious spiritual basis than the other tapping techniques, reflecting Fleming's orientation. You can find information about TAT training at http://www.tatlife.net/resource.

ENERGY MEDICINE

David Feinstein, a clinical psychologist, is married to Donna Eden, the maven of energy medicine. Feinstein has conducted and compiled research studies on many kinds of energy psychology techniques. He and others have developed techniques based on qigong, meditative techniques, martial arts, and other Asian as well as Western practices. These techniques go beyond tapping and include powerful interventions for calming, grounding, and diagnosing emotional and physical distress. Many of Eden's techniques are helpful for clearing energetic blocks to healing. Some can completely clear trauma symptoms. All are safe and helpful for self-use by clients.

One of my favorite of their techniques is the protective "zip up." As I learned it from Wayne McClesky in his 2004 class, you start with both hands a few inches in front of your pubic bone, then raise them straight up to your forehead, three times. This exercise helps direct the flow of the central meridian to armor against other peoples' assaultive or distressing energies.

Other Energy Psychology Resources

Fred Gallo, *Energy Tapping for Trauma: Rapid Relief from Post-Traumatic Stress Using Energy Psychology* (New Harbinger, 2007). Another tapping system with chapters about research and other psychotherapies.

Fred Gallo, *Energy Psychology in Psychotherapy* (Norton, 2002). For professionals.

David Feinstein, Donna Eden, and Gary Craig, *The Promise of Energy Psychology: Revolutionary Tools for Dramatic Personal Change* (Penguin, 2005).

David Feinstein's Web site has many energy psychology resources: http://www.innersource.net/ep

Clinical Wrap-Up

You can cure simple phobias in classically phobic clients in one session using TFT. You can teach energy psychology techniques to your anxiety-disordered clients and complex trauma clients for calming and symptom reduction to use between sessions. When clients flood and lose their ability to stay in the room while confronting overwhelming trauma, use TFT and other energy psychology techniques to quickly reduce the affect overload so that clients can stay with and then clear their traumatic material. When EMDR or ego state work gets stuck, use energy psychology to diagnose and move blocks to processing. It's a valuable tool. It can work.

If you become an energy psychology practitioner, some of your colleagues will likely ridicule you. I've heard from people that it is "woo-woo BS," and that I'm an idiot and performing malpractice for using it. I refer them to the research. I offer to do a session with them. When they're amazed at the results, I refer them to training.

CHAPTER THIRTEEN

Brainspotting & Observed Experiential Integration

David Grand (n.d.), one of the great innovators in EMDR, developed Brainspotting (BSP) as he worked with clients. While BSP isn't backed by EMDR's massive body of research, it is enthusiastically adopted by most who are trained in it. Brainspotting clients listen to CDs with continual bilateral stimulation (BLS) embedded into music, ocean waves, or other sounds, while the therapist uses a pointer to find the "eye spot" that creates a body reaction. Clients experience fast, deep responses and move quickly through issues.

Brainspotting differs from EMDR in several ways:

1. EMDR uses intermittent BLS from one source, while BSP clients wear headsets that play continual BLS, most often from Grand's CDs of music with embedded BLS, while staring at a fixed spot.

2. BSP has a simpler protocol:
   • Activation: Focus on the worst part of the event, problem, or feeling.
   • SUDS: How distressing is it, on a scale of 1 to 10?
   • Body: Where do you feel it in your body?
   • When the client achieves a focused state, turn on the continual BLS.
   • Find the eye spot and hold.

3. Fewer eye movements than EMDR; instead BSP uses a fixed gaze found in one of two ways.
   • In "outside window," the therapist makes a slow sweep with a

wand or pointer and finds the most activated place in the eye. The therapist observes eye blinks, coughs, tics, spasms, or shaking, and holds the wand on the eye spot that creates that response until the distress reaction abates.

- In "inside window," the therapist collaborates with the client to find the spots in the eyes that are the most activated by relying on feedback from the client. The trauma eye and trauma spot are the most activated spots. The resource eye and resource spot are the least activated places.

4. Resourcing is built into regular BSP application. For fragile clients, Grand uses the hypnotic or somatic technique of finding a place that feels "strong, healthy, and grounded," the body resource spot, and holds a resource eye spot on that. Later he "pendulates," going back and forth between the resource and the trauma spots in the eyes and body. Peter Levine (1997) does something similar in his somatic experiencing work.

5. Lisa Schwarz (2008) uses resource spots and an eye spot for each dissociative part in her BSP protocol for dissociative clients. For example, a frightened child part may be stimulated by a focus in the center of the left eye, while an adult part may be found in the top third to the right in the right eye.

6. Brainspotting processing seems to move faster than EMDR processing, but without as many associative connections. This can be more containing for clients with complex trauma and dissociation, causing less flooding.

7. It is possible, but not advised, to do the EMDR protocol by rote, without careful attunement, and still have it work. Since BSP is based on careful attunement and response to clients' slightest responses, an unattuned therapist would most likely fail at using it.

8. BSP doesn't have a careful complete protocol, nor the research and scholarly backup of EMDR. A newer therapy, it is still under construction, with innovations welcome from both trainers and practitioners.

Observed and Experiential Integration (OEI)

Audrey Cook and Rick Bradshaw's OEI, formerly known as the "One Eye Technique" is similar to Brainspotting, in its emphasis on ocular phenomena, sensation, and affect. OEI clients focus on a traumatic event while covering one eye at a time and noticing the difference between the experiences of seeing through each eye. Trauma processing may involve continually covering one eye then the other, going back and forth until the trauma clears, or keeping the more reactive eye open while stimulating the "glitch," leading tiny eye movements across the part of the eye that "jumps" when stimulated. Cook and Bradshaw say that their technique works as quickly as EMDR, but is less distressing to clients who have complex trauma, preventing flooding and dissociative reactions.

CLINICAL WRAP-UP

Brainspotting is a fast, intense, and attuned trauma therapy. If you are an experienced attuned therapist, who understands dissociation, you can add it to your toolbox. If you're starting out, I'd suggest getting the EMDR training first to have the breadth and depth of research, organizations, and a comprehensive therapy under your belt before you learn BSP.

Brainspotting Resources

Visit http://www.brainspotting.pro for training resources and additional information.

OEI Resources

Visit http://www.sightpsychology.com for information on OEI and OEI research, and to order client handbooks and clinician manuals.

CHAPTER FOURTEEN

Reenactment Protocol

Jim Cole's reenactment protocol (RP) combines elements of somatic therapy, imaginal work, hypnotherapy, and some bilateral stimulation. Cole says that "the RP is a process of developing a new active image that reflects control, safety and efficacy that is then associated with the trauma to allow the client a new set of meanings" (2005, p. 212). And it's the only therapy either he or I have done that tends to end with a giggle. Cole says to use the RP with single-trauma events during which the clients were inactive or helpless. It seems to take clients from the freeze or shutdown action/emotional systems into a sense of power and adequacy, sometimes in minutes.

RP TRAUMA PROTOCOL

Here's how it goes:

1. Have the client think of a traumatic event and rate it for amount of distress.

2. Explain the process to the client. In Cole's words: "Fantasies and dreams seem to have a powerful influence. You have likely had some dreams where you woke up with a strong feeling and recalled having things happen in the dream that weren't physically possible. Even when these things were clearly not possible, you still experienced the feelings. Let's use this process with bilateral stimulation in order to have more access to some emotions and recovery. Imagine yourself being unlimited by the laws

of the physical world. You are able to do superhuman things. Imagine that you can reach long distances, exert great forces, move with lightning speed and generally do any superhuman task. With these powers, go back to the time of the trauma or just before the trauma and create a new memory or story. In doing this, take note of the pain you have experienced and imagine yourself fully using that part of your body in this superhuman fantasy with powerful physical strength in that part of your body. I want you to decide what you will do, then share it with me" (2005, p. 216).

3. Cole advises clients to use the present tense, with a personal and active voice. The imaginal reenactment occurs in a here and now in which the client takes control and dominates the situation, feels safe, is active, and uses the limb or body part that was hurt or holds the sensation of the trauma. He says it's important to give the client time, listen to the new story, ask clarifying questions and give suggestions if needed, and support the superhuman story without criticism. He encourages physical involvement and then focus on sensations during the active process.

4. "Okay, now that you have re-created the incident with you having superhuman powers, I want you to go slowly through this process while we do some bilateral stimulation. I will give you all the time you need. You let me know when you have finished your fantasy."

5. Continue until the client signals that the fantasy is finished. Cole writes: "As the story unfolds I periodically direct the client's attention to the physical sensations and encourage positive feelings of self-appreciation and self-efficacy. I do this by simple reflective statements that direct the client's attention: 'Let yourself feel the strength in your arm as you reach out and stop the oncoming car.' Or as it was with one client, 'Let yourself feel the strength in your arms, shoulders and back as you resist those who hurt you and take charge of the situation.' With another client I suggested, 'Focus on the strength in your back as you lift that SUV and throw it into orbit'" (2005, p. 217).

6. Note any change in affect. Many clients will laugh or express enjoyment on turning the tables on abuse or an oncoming car.

7. Direct clients to focus on how the superhuman fantasy has changed his or her self-identity. Cole says, "This image of the self then becomes a positive cognition that is referenced in response to the reworked superhuman fantasy. While focusing upon this self-perception I do a few sets of eye movements, or other form of bilateral stimulation, until the feelings seem more true or believable. I often suggest that the client wanted to do those powerful and positive things" (2005, p. 218).

RP TREATMENT EXAMPLES

Car Accident

A woman whose car was T-boned by a drunk driver was afraid to drive again. She was an engaging, well-attached, not otherwise traumatized person, no longer physically hurt a month after the accident, but having flashbacks and anxiety. We did the RP in one session and had one positive follow-up phone call. After explaining the setup, I asked her to bring up the moment right before the impact, and to tell me where she felt the distress in her body. She responded, "Everywhere." I told her, "Take that feeling and use it to fuel you rescuing yourself." She became Super Bouncer and, with her whole body, saw the other car coming and, while pumping up and down in her chair, imagined bouncing her car up in the air over the other car. She laughed hard and imagined bouncing her car on her errands for the rest of what had been the day of the accident, still laughing. She was completely over the accident in that one session.

Organized Rape of a Child

The client said, "I imagined growing very long and thin and slippery so I could slip out of the ties. Then I pretended I was VERY strong and I stood up on the bed with my back to the wall and I shouted very loud STOP!! And I kept shouting STOP till all the grown-ups in the room got very small. Then I scooped them up and put them in a little wooden box and gave them to the police to take care of" (Cole, 2005, p. 220).

Traumatic Grief

See Chapter 23 for another example of RP.

For Chronic Pain Connected With a Traumatic Event

Cole says, "It's important that the guided image be related to the specific body parts that were involved in the original trauma. The best image is the one that the client identifies with most easily. . . . Attention is given to the same motor centers that were involved in the original accident or pain incident in order to stimulate the same motor centers and both create new strength associations and weaken existing pain associations. For this reason use the same muscles in the reenactment fantasy that originally generated the signals to the brainstem motor centers" (2005, p. 224).

RP Pain Example

Another car accident: A therapist in Cole's RP workshop had a sore leg months after ramming her car into the abruptly stopping car ahead of her. I saw Cole do the setup, having her focus on the sensations in her sore leg. He told her to find a way to use that leg in her fantasy. She became Rubber Woman, with her powerful elastic leg pushing into the stopped car, absorbing the shock and cushioning the cars so they didn't hit. Within minutes she was smiling, and her leg stopped hurting, for good.

Summary

The RP is effective with physically based, single-event trauma. It can relieve trauma-based pain. It's often fun for the client and for the therapist. It doesn't appear to cause abreactions. It's fast, with most interventions taking under 10 minutes.

Resources

Find the full RP protocol in Jim Cole, "The Reenactment Protocol," in R. Shapiro (Ed.), *EMDR Solutions: Pathways to Healing* (Norton, 2005, pp. 8–56).

CHAPTER FIFTEEN

David Grove's Trauma Therapy

David Grove did a very directed kind of exposure therapy (Grove & Panzer, 1989). As the client would start to tell the story of the trauma, Grove would repeat what she said in a ritualized way, using her language, but in the present tense to move the story along. He thought that trauma survivors were often stuck at the beginning or in the middle of a traumatic event and needed to be moved forward to the end, when it was over and they were safe. He would instruct clients to tell him the story of the trauma and would repeat back exactly what they said in a very particular protocol. Notice how this technique moves the story forward.

Client: And then I heard him coming up the stairs.

Therapist: He's coming up the stairs. He's coming up the stairs. What happens next when he's coming up the stairs?

Client: He walks into my room and sits on the bed.

Therapist: He's sitting on the bed. He's sitting on the bed. What happens next when he's sitting on the bed?

Client: He pulls the covers down.

Therapist: He pulls the covers down. He pulls the covers down. What happens next when he pulls the covers down?

Client: I freeze.

Therapist: You freeze. You freeze. And for how long do you freeze, and what happens next?

I'll skip the gory parts here and go to the end. Notice how the use of the present tense increases the immediacy of the statements and moves the story forward. Using Grove's method, you both follow and lead the client through the trauma until it's over:

Client: He covers me up and goes away.

Therapist: He goes away. He goes away. And what happens next when he goes away?

Client: I cry myself to sleep.

Therapist: You cry yourself to sleep, you sleep, and for how long do you sleep and what happens next?

Client: I get up and take a bath and have breakfast and go to school.

Clients are contained by the ritual and brought through the trauma to the end. This containing, relational exposure technique was my most effective trauma tool until I learned EMDR in the mid-1990s. Still, when a current client is stuck in a memory without good dual attention, unable to feel herself in the room, or is beginning to dissociate, I use Grove's powerful "What happens next?" technique to put them back onto the mindful, present track.

I've had clients who had died and then been revived and others who had been trapped in horrible abuse situations. Grove's technique got the memories unstuck from the moment of death or the worst moment of the abuse with dialogue like this:

- You're dead. You're dead. And for how long are you dead? And what happens next when you're dead?
- You're trapped. You're trapped. And for how long are you trapped? And what happens next when you're trapped?
- He's beating [raping, smothering] you. He's beating you. And what happens next when he's beating you?
- You're feeling helpless. You're feeling helpless. And for how long do you feel helpless? And what happens next when you're helpless?

RESOURCE

David J. Grove and B. I. Panzer, *Resolving Traumatic Memories* (Irvington, 1989).

CHAPTER SIXTEEN

Neurofeedback

Neurofeedback is a form of biofeedback that teaches the brain to become more calm and even. At its best, neurofeedback improves sleep, relaxation, and mental acuity. In quantitative EEG and alpha theta brainwave neurofeedback, clients either watch a computer screen with a simple game on it or respond to tones while wearing sensors that detect specific brainwave activities. Through the cues, they can detect when their brains approach optimal settings, which they do by moving the "beta" spaceship up or creating more "good" tones. It's an operant conditioning exercise that works well. As their brain waves approach the desired state, they are rewarded by a visual or aural cue. Gradually, they are trained to bring their brains into line with optimum functioning. In nonentrainment neurofeedback (Doerfler, 2009), subtle cues tell clients when their brain waves are out of sync. "In Low Energy Neurofeedback Systems (LENS) a machine tracks what's happening in the brain and answers it with a radio wave that 'nudges' the brain. LENS is not learning, it's a passive intervention" (Emily Elliot, personal communication, November 6, 2009). Early studies showed that neurofeedback works to abate PTSD in veterans (Peniston & Kulkosky, 1991, 1992). More recently, neuropsychiatrist and researcher Bessel van der Kolk has found it useful with highly dissociated people and has incorporated a neurofeedback component into his clinic for further research. Emily Elliot, a Seattle practitioner, says that with neurofeedback, "traumatized and other people's brain function improve[s]. They become more lucid and functional and perform daily tasks with more ease. They have better impulse control and improved self awareness" (personal communication, November 6, 2009).

This is what I noticed with one client who did several months of LENS after 6 years of intensive therapy for DID, depression, and intractable physical flashback symptoms. Before neurofeedback, he had become functional, able to work again, able to successfully parent his children and to be a good friend. However, he was still horribly symptomatic and became flooded with any attempt to deal directly with the horrors of his childhood. After neurofeedback, he became more coherent when speaking about his past and much more able to hold the dual attention (awareness of now, while thinking about back then) that is necessary for trauma therapy. He could tolerate his body sensations without regression. He showed less anxiety. Current events that would have triggered him into self-injury or extreme suicidal ideation still bothered him, but didn't cause harm. He began to write about his experiences in a deeply philosophical way, an activity that formerly would have flooded him with flashbacks and awful sensations. Because of these changes, especially in coherency, we were able to shorten our 90-minute sessions to 60 minutes. Our work continues, more quickly and more fruitfully.

Neurofeedback Resources

John Demos, *Getting Started With Neurofeedback* (Norton, 2004).

Jim Robbins, *A Symphony in the Brain: The Evolution of the New Brain Wave Biofeedback* (Grove, 2008).

"Neurofeedback (EEG Biofeedback) Provides Alternative Approach to Post-Traumatic Stress Disorder (PTSD)." A comprehensive online article with many good references, available at http://www.growing.com/mind/PTSD/index.htm

CHAPTER SEVENTEEN

Medications

Trauma is a physical phenomenon. PTSD continually recreates the bodily reactions of the original distressing moments: the unmyelinated part of the vagal nerve turns on, the limbic system lights up, respiration and heart rate change to support flight or fight, and stress hormones release, "such that traumatic memories become overconsolidated, easily activated, and overwhelming in their capacity to produce negative emotions" (Scott & Briere, 2006, p. 190). PTSD and long-term abuse and neglect can change the brain, reducing the size of the hippocampus (Perry, 2000) and suppressing cortisol production (Hart, Gunnar, & Cicchetti, 1995), creating biological states of depression, anxiety, pain, and digestive difficulties, to name a few.

Medical interventions including medications, neurofeedback, and acupuncture work directly on the body to allay or mediate the symptoms of PTSD.

Medications don't cure PTSD or the nervous system changes from early or long-term trauma. Medications can ease symptoms, bringing clients inside the window of tolerance, not too flooded or too shut down, so that psychotherapeutic interventions can work. Trauma survivors who avoid or don't have access to psychotherapy may use medications for long-term symptom relief. This chapter includes the most common medications used in treatment of trauma symptoms.

Prazosin

Prazosin (Minipress, Vasoflex, Hypovase) is an old blood pressure drug that has been found to eliminate or lessen nightmares, improve sleep, and sometimes lessen other PTSD symptoms in trauma survivors. It's inexpensive, has few side effects, is not sedating, is not addictive, and allows normal dreaming. It was first prescribed for and studied with Veterans Administration clients (Raskind et al., 2003) and has since been used for civilian patients (Taylor & Raskind, 2002). Some of my clients have found it useful for sleeping without nightmares.

ANTIDEPRESSANTS

Antidepressants are the most prescribed medications for PTSD and DESNOS clients. Selective serotonin reuptake inhibitors (SSRIs) are the most prescribed antidepressants. They may lighten moods, decrease anxiety, decrease obsessive thoughts, and decrease specific PTSD symptoms such as flashbacks. Many clients resist taking them, saying, "If I'm taking medication, that means I'm really crazy," or, "I don't want to deal with the side effects." Side effects can include "anxiety, nervousness, sweating, headache, gastrointestinal upset (nausea, diarrhea, dyspepsia), dry mouth, somnolence, insomnia, and disruption of all phases of sexuality (erections in men, and libido and orgasms in both men and women)" (Scott & Briere, 2006, p. 199). When people on SSRIs quit them abruptly, rather than tapering off, they may experience discontinuation syndrome, including muscle twitches, the sense of electric shock, sleeplessness, inability to eat, tremor, stomach problems, and severe anxiety.

Common SSRIs include fluoxetine (Prozac), fluvoxamine (Luvox), citalopram (Celexa), paroxetine (Paxil), sertraline (Zoloft) and escitalopram (Lexapro). Clients who take SSRIs can have reduced PTSD symptoms of reexperiencing, hyperarousal, and avoidance. They may sleep better, have a lighter mood, and more hope. They often are better able to make use of therapy, neither too hyperaroused or hypoaroused to tolerate thinking about their traumas. They may see improved function in much of their lives.

Bessel van der Kolk and his cohorts did a groundbreaking study on the effects of EMDR treatment versus Prozac versus a placebo pill control group in traumatized depressed people:

> Eighty-eight PTSD subjects diagnosed according to DSM-IV criteria were randomly assigned to EMDR, fluoxetine, or pill placebo. They received 8 weeks of treatment and were assessed by blind raters posttreat-

ment and at 6-month follow-up. The primary outcome measure was the Clinician-Administered PTSD Scale, DSM-IV version, and the secondary outcome measure was the Beck Depression Inventory-II. The study ran from July 2000 through July 2003. RESULTS: The psychotherapy intervention was more successful than pharmacotherapy in achieving sustained reductions in PTSD and depression symptoms, but this benefit accrued primarily for adult-onset trauma survivors. At 6-month follow-up, 75.0% of adult-onset versus 33.3% of child-onset trauma subjects receiving EMDR achieved asymptomatic end-state functioning compared with none in the fluoxetine group. (van der Kolk et al., 2007)

Got that? With 8 weeks of therapy, 75% had no symptoms of PTSD or depression versus 0% losing all their symptoms after 8 weeks of Prozac. Adult-onset subjects tended to improve for months after their EMDR treatments, and stayed that way. Van der Kolk's team felt that with more than 8 weeks of treatment the child-onset PTSD group could have had much better results. Some studies have shown that treating PTSD with SSRIs for at least 9 months could lead to longer term lessening or cessation of some symptoms (Davidson, 2004).

SSRIs are the most widely used antidepressants. Older medications, the tricylics and MAO inhibitors, have even worse side effects. Newer medications related to SSRIs include venlafaxine (Effexor), mirtazapine (Remeron), trazodone (Desyrel), nefazodone (Serzone), and bupropion (Wellbutrin). Some are more sedating. Some are more activating. Some have different side effects in different people. And all antidepressants should be prescribed by a doctor or nurse practitioner with a thorough knowledge of the benefits and risks of each medication.

BENZODIAZEPINES

Right after a trauma, survivors may display panic attacks, agitation, and insomnia. They may be in acute distress and want to do or take anything to become calm and normal again. Benzodiazepines will often bring calm and sleep to the most agitated person. They include alprazolam (Xanax), clonazepam (Klonopin), diazepam (Valium), lorazepam (Ativan), temazepam (Restoril), triazolam (Halcion), and oxazepam (Serax). There's a catch: All benzodiazepines are highly addictive. Many patients develop tolerance to them and have to take more and more to achieve the same calming affect. They work on almost everyone but are hell to get off. I've had clients who had to taper off by fractions of a milligram every few weeks to quit these drugs. Each time they took less, they had to endure acute anxiety, and sometimes anxiety attacks, for several days. As a nonmedical practitioner, I see three trauma-related uses for benzodiazepines:

1. As a short-acting stop to the worst panic attacks, taken as needed

2. As an occasional sleep aid, if nothing else works

3. As a remedy immediately after the traumatic event, so that the client can regain a sense of control

According to Scott and Briere, "Regular use of benzodiazepines may interfere with the processing of traumatic material in therapy, or may produce state-dependent treatment effects that do not persist once medication has been discontinued" (2006, p. 208). Francine Shapiro agrees: "the benzodiazepines have been reported to reduce treatment efficacy [with EMDR] with some clients" (2001, p. 102). She recommends reprocessing the traumatic events, if needed, after clients have stopped taking the medication.

OPIATE ANTAGONISTS

When people who are traumatized as adults are reexposed to situations reminiscent of the trauma, it increases their endogenous (internally generated) opioids (Gold, Pottash, Sweeney, Martin, & Extein, 1982). People who were abused or neglected in their early years may have a long-term endogenous opioid reaction, chronic dissociation. They may be less sensitive to pain, lethargic, more rigid or more flaccid, and essentially immobile. Ulrich Lanius (2005) has found that the opiate antagonists that block both endogenous and exogamous (from the outside) opiates can help highly dissociated people in two ways: (1) administered right before a session, the medications can help clients stay in the room with dual attention so that they can bear holding traumatic events in mind without switching, flooding, or shutting down; (2) taken as a daily medication, they reduce dissociative symptoms (Schmahl, Stiglmayr, Böhme, & Bohus, 1999) including "tonic immobility, analgesia, and flashbacks" (Bohus et al., 1999).

A small group of therapists and medicators are using injectable naloxone (Narcan, Nalone, Narcanti) or naltrexone (Revia, Depade) pills with borderline, DDNOS, and DID clients. Many of them find that clients are more able to tolerate remembering and clearing traumatic events. Clients who take daily doses are less prone to flashbacks, less triggered into dissociative states, and more present overall.

RESOURCES

Catherine Scott and John Briere, "Biology and Psychopharmacology of Trauma" in J. Briere and C. Scott (Eds.), *Principles of Trauma Therapy: A Guide to Symptoms, Evaluation, and Treatment* (Sage, 2006). One of the most understandable discussions of the whys and hows of psychotropic medication for trauma.

Ulrich Lanius, "EMDR Processing With Dissociative Clients: Adjunctive Use of Opioid Antagonists," in R. Shapiro (Ed.), *EMDR Solutions: Pathways to Healing* (Norton, 2005). It gives research, theory, and dosages. I've given the chapter to psychiatrists, who then prescribed the correct dosages to my clients. And they were fascinated.

Many Web sites and books exist, for laypeople, helping professionals, and prescribers.

Part IV

THERAPIES FOR
COMPLEX TRAUMA

Most trauma therapies have at least partial results with single-episode traumas, when clients have good attachment and subsequent good affect tolerance and have had no previous big traumas. Unfortunately, most people who consult therapists have more complex trauma. As you have read in Chapters 1 and 2, traumatic experiences have effects ranging from, "it was scary and awful but I'm over it" to full-blown dissociative identity disorder. In this section you will find chapters about:

1. Attachment-based trauma

2. Ego state therapies

3. Treatment for all levels of complex trauma with the structural dissociation model

4. Treatment for borderline personality disorder, including Linehan's dialectical behavior therapy

In Christine Courtois and Julian Ford's excellent edited book, Treating Complex Traumatic Stress Disorders, they define "complex psychological trauma as involving traumatic stressors that (1) are repetitive or prolonged; (2) involve direct harm and/or neglect and abandonment by caregivers or ostensibly responsible adults; (3) occur at developmentally vulnerable times in the victim's life, such as early childhood; and (4) have great potential to compromise severely a child's development" (2009, p. 1).

Judith Herman, the godmother of healing relational trauma, wrote the foreword for the book, noticing that most of its authors agreed that clinicians should "recognize areas of strength and resilience" in their clients, develop a "trusting and truly collaborative, rather than authoritarian, treatment relationship," just as clients need to develop that sort of mindful trust inside themselves, growing into the ability to self-soothe. She also noted that most therapies for complex trauma have three stages: establishing safety, coming to terms with the trauma, and repairing and enlarging the survivor's social connections.

CHAPTER EIGHTEEN

The Trauma of Disrupted Attachment

Many traumas are dramatic and obvious. Rapes, bad accidents, battle-fields, cataclysms, and violence cause obvious trauma and, often, PTSD. Much of what we treat is less dramatic, but no less disruptive. Poor or disrupted attachment, which can be developmentally devastating, may come from small, subtle, often repeated interactions. Edward Tronick (2007) showed how a mother's still, unresponsive face could take a baby or toddler from happily connected to frantic, to shut down, in a matter of minutes. Imagine a baby with a chronically depressed, addicted, or distressed caregiver. Depending on the developmental window during which a child has an inconsistent, unresponsive, or frightening caregiver, she or he may not learn to connect, self-regulate, identify feeling states, experience a baseline of safety, or know herself or himself to be a valuable, lovable person (Schore, 1994; Siegel, 1999). Some children are raised with constitutionally anxious parents, or angry parents, or with too many other kids around to get adequate attention. And others are born into refugee families or bad neighborhoods, or to parents with unhealed trauma whose anxiety was always in the air. These children absorb the anxiety around them, as if deep into their bones.

People with disrupted early attachment may have these problems:

- An inconsistent sense of self
- Trouble identifying feelings and wants
- Poor affect regulation
- Low self-esteem, to the point of holding themselves to be worth-less

- Depression
- Poor relational skills, including lack of assertiveness
- Either volatile or low-intimacy relationships or no relationships
- Either overresponsibility or no ability to feel responsible in relational conflicts
- Codependence, putting everyone else's needs first
- Dissociation

Infants who are subject to chronic relational disconnect learn to shut down. It is possible for attachment trauma alone, with no obvious physical or sexual abuse, to create high levels of lifelong dissociation (Liotti, 2006). Liotti found:

1. Pathological dissociation is relational and hinders the integrative processes of consciousness, rather than being an intrapsychic defense against mental pain.

2. "Early defenses against attachment-related dissociation are based on interpersonal controlling strategies that inhibit the attachment system." (p. 55)

3. Dissociative symptoms emerge as a consequence of the collapse of these defensive strategies in the face of events that powerfully activate the attachment system.

4. Psychotherapy of attachment with disturbed or dissociative clients "should be a phase-oriented process focused primarily on achieving attachment security, and only secondarily on trauma work." (p. 55)

Attachment therapy has three stages:

1. A strong, trusting, intersubjective therapeutic relationship with the first focus on healing the attachment injuries
2. Clearing of the trauma and shame
3. Skill building to create better relationships

GOOD THERAPIES FOR HEALING ATTACHMENT DEFICITS

Psychodynamic: No matter what other modality you use, you must use the therapeutic relationship as an anchor, a mirror, and an engine for repair of dissociated and attachment-impaired clients. Elements of

Diana Fosha's accelerated experiential-dynamic psychotherapy or any other active and containing psychodynamic therapies let you intervene immediately in dysfunctional interactions. Use yourself to create interpersonal safety and intersubjectivity (you and the client knowing that you are sharing the same emotional experience at the same time), and to induce the sense of being delightful in your client.

Ego state therapies: Inside every adult with poor attachment is a child part who didn't have his or her needs met. All of the ego state therapies give templates to meet the needs of the younger parts, buoy the adult parts, and bring integration to the whole. The bigger the attachment deficit, the more likely you will have a dissociated client and will need to use ego state therapy.

EMDR: Maureen Kitchur's (2005) strategic developmental model for EMDR suggests you have the attachment-disordered client imagine looking up into her mother's or other caregiver's eyes as an infant, and target the affect and sensations the client feels in this moment. When that distress clears, you have the client imagine the scenario as a toddler, then a grade schooler, with mom responding in her typical way (looking away, looking distracted, angry, sad, overwhelmed, etc.), then clear what arises with EMDR. Brainspotting works well on the same targets.

Somatic psychotherapies: Sensorimotor psychotherapy and somatic transformation combine attention to attachment, sensory experience, and movement to help heal attachment injuries and grow vibrant, connected people.

Skill building: If clients had early attachment injuries, they may not know how to interact authentically, assertively, and for their own good. The last part of the therapy will involve learning new interpersonal skills and bringing them into the world.

Simple exposure and simple cognitive therapies: These therapies may retraumatize and frustrate people with deep-seated attachment issues. Go for relational bottom-up therapies to heal attachment injuries. Read about dialectical behavior therapy in Chapter 21 for a cognitive behavior therapy that is suited to attachment-based trauma.

CLEARING AN ATTACHMENT-BASED DEPRESSION

I'm using a high-functioning client in this example. You may use the same tools with more distressed and neglected clients.

Jean is a retired helping professional in her 60s. She's intelligent, sensitive, anxious, and depressed. She wants to feel better, heal the wounds of a failed relationship, and know who she is. She'd like less anxiety and more energy and pleasure. At the intake, we found a middle-class Southern family. Mom was narcissistic. Dad mostly gone. The culture of the small town bred conformity and inhibition, especially in its female members. In one of her first memories, Jean was 2, sitting on the kitchen floor, playing with baking pans. Her mother rushed into the room, yelling, "We don't play on the floor. That's for trash!" Mom didn't connect with Jean and was either oblivious to her or overinvolved with Jean's appearance. Jean was molested by a neighbor boy. She was continually shamed by her older sister. She grew up charming on the outside and empty on the inside. She has been married and divorced, but no relationship ever sustained her. She has friends, but isn't often "real" with them.

The Relationship

Jean had the kind of personality that is fast to connect, but fast to feel hurt, which makes for a quick start in therapy. We talked about her attachment deficits and how important it was for us to keep our relationship in good repair. We talked about not doing trauma work until she felt safe. Jean compulsively took care of everyone, including me. I'd tease her when she'd try: "Honey [she was Southern and we were both female, so I could call her Honey], do you think I would adore you less if you didn't try to take care of me?" She would giggle and go back to her work. As the relationship deepened over the weeks, she would talk about how good it felt to be seen and accepted and to see that her hurts and growth affected me. In the later months of therapy, we often laughed together and high-fived with each triumph.

Clearing Trauma

When we both felt ready, we cleared the molestation memory in three sessions of EMDR. Then we went after Mom.

Therapist: You're an infant in your mother's arms. Look up at her face. What do you see?

Jean: It's like a mask.

Therapist: When you look into that mask, what do you say to your-self about yourself?

Jean: I'm not okay. . . . In fact, I'm not . . . here.

Therapist: What's the opposite?

Jean: I am here. I exist!

Therapist: When you're a baby, looking into your mom's face, how true, 1 to 7, does it feel in your gut that you exist?

Jean: Not very true, a 2, maybe.

She felt empty, in her core: emptiness tinged with anxiety. As we processed with EMDR, she went from empty to tense to mad to sad. "I was there. She [Mom] wasn't there! She didn't know what to do. I was okay. I always existed. . . . But I really didn't have a mother." She expressed sad affect and tears. We did several more rounds of processing. Finally, spontaneously and strongly, she said, "I deserved to have a mother who was there and I didn't have one."

I said, "Go with that!" We finished the session with installing the idea, "I exist and I deserve attention." When we were done, the petite woman seemed a head taller. As homework, Jean listened to April Steele's imaginal nurturing tapes (see Chapter 19) every day for 2 weeks, and learned to nurture and find delight in her own infant and toddler selves.

We targeted the kitchen floor incident, then did five sessions of other interactions with her mother. Jean realized that the molestation and an incident of being stuck on a roof were due, in part, to her mother's inattention. She began to see her mother's internalized pressure to conform, as a Southern woman, as an inheritance from her mother's family. Jean saw her mother's competition with her for her father's scant attention. The more she cleared, the more she knew: "It wasn't about me. It was about who my mother was. I was okay and I'm still okay." Jean began to move through anger and sadness near the end of each session as she realized how her family's dynamic squelched her aliveness. As we processed through the grief, she always came to this idea: "But I can be different now." And we always installed it.

As the trauma left, we brought more focus to the body: "What do you feel in your body now? What posture would express that? Great! Strike a pose! You're looking grown up and strong to me. What does it feel like when you hold your body like that?"

Identifying Wants

If you can't know what you want, it's hard to know who you are. We started with a simple forced-choice exercise that helped Jean identify how to know what she wanted.

Therapist: Okay, Jean, right now what appeals the most: chocolate or vanilla?

Jean: Vanilla.

Therapist: Where do you feel that in your body?

Jean: My tongue and my stomach.

We continued through questions like romantic comedies versus slasher movies, coffee versus tea, men versus women, and different social situations and locations. Jean's assignment that week was to notice her body's reaction to several choices each day: food, activities, and especially processing requests from others. She noticed that she became more decisive and more assertive after a few weeks of practicing conscious choosing.

Skills

The depression lifted as Jean began to experience weekly epiphanies. "I've reorganized my house so that it's comfortable for me, not for how it looks. I've bought a big comfortable chair for me. I may never let anyone else sit on it. It's my throne. I'm the queen of my house." Other weeks she talked about how her social life was shifting. Sessions become more oriented to the present, to bringing new skills into her current life. I would make ridiculous requests and she would practice saying no to me. We would discuss strategy for dealing with needy or dismissive friends and her sick and still narcissistic mother.

Jean's mother needed help to close down the family home and move into assisted living. Before Jean flew out of state to help her mother, we had two future-pacing, skill-oriented sessions. We strategized and then practiced what she would do.

Jean: I'm afraid that I'll be totally absorbed into my mother's needs.

Therapist: You're there. Imagine the space. Your mother is distressed and relentless. What are you saying to yourself about yourself?

Jean: I can't say no. I have to do everything. I'm not enough.

Therapist: What do you want to say?

Jean: I have limits and can enforce them. . . . I have choices.

Therapist: So let's run through how you can exercise those choices. How can you set it up from the beginning? You're a highly sensitive introvert. How do you take care of that kind of person?

Jean: I'll need breaks from my mother. I'll need to walk every day. I'll need to have regular meals. And I shouldn't stay in the chaotic house, because it would drive me crazy.

Therapist: Great. How would you set that up? [She talks about the details, and tells me that the worst part will be telling her mother about her plans to stay elsewhere.] When you think about telling your mom, how big is the anxiety?

Jean: Six out of 10, in my throat.

Therapist: Go with that. [EMDR with BLS.]

Jean: It's going down fast. A 2. [BLS] . . . I do have a choice, even if it makes me nervous. It's hard to say no to my mom. [BLS] I can do it. I have to take care of myself.

Therapist: Great. I want you to run through the phone call and your mom's likely reactions. Then we'll run through a bunch of scenarios that are likely to occur when you're there. Start with the phone call. Imagine dialing the phone to tell your mom that you're not staying at the house during the move.

Jean: I can do it. I feel resolved. [BLS]

Jean moved through that and several scenarios involving her mother, the amount of work to do, family members, and other people. We used BLS on any twinges of anxiety, which became less and less as she progressed through the various tasks and scenarios of the trip. When she returned from the trip, she was triumphant. She had opportunities to stand her ground, and she did. Mostly, she noticed what she needed, took care of herself, and stayed reasonably calm and grounded throughout the trip.

After a full year of therapy, Jean has no depression, has kept only the friends who support her, and is engaged in a full and happy retirement. She is using her newfound skills to find herself a "keeper," a man who can be a match for her vitality and assertiveness.

ATTACHMENT RESOURCES

Dan Siegel and Marion Solomon (Eds.), *Healing Trauma: Attachment, Mind, Body, and Brain* (Norton, 2003). It's got all the big names in trauma and attachment and is a great overview.

Dan Siegel, *The Developing Mind: How Relationships and the Brain Interact to Shape Who We Are* (Guilford, 2001). An important explanation of how attachment affects the brain. An amazing book.

Louis Cozolino, *The Neuroscience of Psychotherapy: Building and Rebuilding the Human Brain* (Norton, 2002).

Thomas Lewis, Fari Amini, and Richard Lannon, *A General Theory of Love* (Vintage, 2001). A poetic, brief, user-friendly book about attachment that, despite having nothing good to say about trauma therapy, must be read by everyone.

David Wallin, *Attachment in Psychotherapy* (Guilford, 2007).

Diana Fosha, *The Transforming Power of Affect: A Model for Accelerated Change* (Basic Books, 2000). No matter what kind of therapy you do, if you read this book, you'll do it better. Great information about attachment, affect, and how to do good therapy.

CHAPTER NINETEEN

Ego State Therapies

Therapist: Check inside. What age is that voice that's telling you that you have to let your boyfriend continue to abuse you?

Client: "She's 4. And she's standing in front of my dad, about to be whipped, because she knows she's bad and deserves it.

Therapist: Can you take that 4-year-old by the hand and start flying her up the years to right here and right now?

Client: Okay.

Therapist: Show her all the milestones. Going to grade school. Junior high. Graduating high school and leaving the house. College. Your jobs. Your marriage. Your daughter growing up. Moving into your current wonderful house (Pace, 2007). [She nods at each one.] And right up to right now in this office. [Nods.] You hold that 4-year-old on your lap. Can you feel her warmth and her weight? Can she feel your strong arms around her as she looks up into your 50-year-old eyes (Steele, 2007)? Show her around your current life: your agency, your house, your grown-up loving daughter, and your three closest friends. Let her know that you've got what it takes to take care of her. Do you agree to take care of her as well as you took care of your daughter?

Client: Yes.

Therapist: Will you make sure that that inside little girl is nutritiously fed, has rest, and is safe at all times? Will you make sure that she's protected from exploitation?

Client: Well, I want to, but she doesn't think she deserves it. Anyway, she loves him.

Therapist: Of course she does. I bet he feels just like Dad.

Client: Oh God, he does!

Therapist: Let me ask you: Do you think it's appropriate for a 4-year-old part of you to run your love life?

Client: Not really.

Therapist: Is it time to lay her off from that grown-up job?

Client: Yeah [resignedly].

Therapist: I want you to notice that little girl's yearning feeling toward that guy. Really feel it. And then I want you to turn her around toward you to look into your eyes. Got it? Good. Tell her that you are the one that's going to be there for her all the time. . . . Tell her that you're the one that can take care of her and hold her and make sure she's safe. . . . And now remind her to notice that you and she are stuck together and that she will always be with you and you will always be with her. Let her know that you will take care of all the grown-up stuff from here on. Does she get it? How do you know?

Client: She's relaxing and snuggling into me. It's like I've taken her back from him.

Therapist: Great! So she knows she lives with you and it's now and she doesn't have to run everything anymore?

Client: Yes!

Therapist: How does that feel?

Client: For the first time, I feel like an adult. I'm 50, but I have never felt like it before.

Therapist: What's it mean to be 50?

Client: I don't have to please everyone anymore. I can take care of myself. I'm safe. And I'm in charge.

Therapist: Wow! What would a grown-up, in-charge woman do with an abusive, manipulative man?

Client: Boot him.

Therapist: What does the 4-year-old think about that?

Client: She's okay. She's with me.

Therapist: Have you hugged her inside already?

Client: She's already inside.

Therapist: Where does she live inside of you?

Client: In my heart.

Ego States

Most of us have ego states, those bundles of neurons that manifest different moods, behaviors, and reactions depending on the demands of our external and internal environments. Think about yourself playing a game, driving on a familiar road, working with a difficult client, doing your shopping, walking into a party where you don't know anyone, or arguing with your beloved. Each of these situations calls forth a different set of reactions, a slightly (or maybe vastly) different response to your inner and outer situation. If you had a benign, well-supported childhood and later life, your ego states, or parts, "live in the present; feel and manage the full range of emotions; hold positive beliefs about self and world; engage in appropriate behaviors; and have an adaptive point of view" (Schmidt, 2009, p. 18) and are likely tied to ages and activities. "Every time I play with the dog, I revert to my 8-year-old self." "I always feel like a teenager when I walk into a party." "As soon as I sit down in my office chair, I become 'the therapist.' When I leave the office, I lose about 20 years of authority and responsibility." You probably can transition smoothly from one state to the other. And you remember things that you said and did in one state, when you are in another. When a threatening or distressing situation arises, the action systems of flight, flee, or cling are available to you, but are neural pathways, not hardened superhighways of rigid reaction.

Dissociative States

A client who was abused or neglected as a child might have dissociative emotional parts that would involve well-trodden wide action (structural dissociation) or emotional (affect theory; Panksepp, 1998) systems that may be fast to fire, intense in expression, and disconnected from adult problem solving and current reality. In some cases, particularly involving severe and chronic abuse and neglect, a client may have several EPs (emotional parts) and ANPs (apparently normal parts), some of which may have strong separate identities and some of which may be mutually amnestic. At any hint or reminder of threat, his brain activates six-lane freeways of reactive selves, parts, or ego states. "Wounded ego states [i.e., dissociative parts] . . . live in the past; are stuck in painful emotions, hold negative, irrational beliefs about self and world; engage in unwanted or inappropriate behaviors; and have a maladaptive point of view" (Schmidt, 2009, p. 18).

EGO STATES VERSUS DISSOCIATIVE STATES

Kathy Steele told me:

Ego states have permeable boundaries, unlike many dissociative parts. They do not involve amnesia, i.e., one ego state is not operating in the outside world without the awareness of another ego state. Ego states do not create "jarring" intrusions into the experience of the person as do dissociative parts. Ego states do not cause a person to experience first-ranked Schneiderian symptoms of schizophrenia: hearing voices commenting or arguing, feeling your body is controlled by someone else; made thoughts, feelings or impulses, etc. They do not have a separate sense of self as dissociative parts do. Ego states experience themselves as the person, albeit perhaps in a different state or age or time. Another way to put it is that dissociative parts have four characteristics that ego states do not: (1) they have their own identities and sense of self; (2) they have a characteristic self-representation, which may not be consistent with the self representation of the individual as whole; (3) they have their own set of autobiographical memories, which may be different than other dissociative parts; (4) they have a sense of ownership of their own thoughts, feelings, actions, etc. A good rule to follow: All dissociative parts are ego states, but not all ego states are dissociative parts. (personal communication, September 19, 2009)

Be aware that when people talk about ego state therapy, they are often talking about dissociative state therapy. Many clinicians use the words interchangeably, so listen carefully. Are they talking about here-and-now, associated parts, or reflexively triggered, dissociated, separate parts?

EGO STATE THERAPY

Ego state therapy works directly with parts of consciousness to create a cohesive, coherent, trauma-healed whole, with flexibility between parts and appropriate responses to here and now. It's the embodiment of dual attention, the ability to hold onto present consciousness while remembering traumatic states. Ego state therapy, alone or combined with other therapies, is a powerful tool for working with most survivors of chronic childhood abuse and neglect. It is a necessary part of therapy with every DID client.

Emmerson stated that the goals of ego state therapy are as follows:

1) to locate ego states [dissociative parts] harboring pain, trauma, anger, or frustration, and facilitate expression, release, comfort, and empowerment;
2) to facilitate functional communication among the ego states; and
3) to help clients learn their ego states so that the states may better be used to the clients' benefit. (2003, p. x)

In this chapter you'll read about several ways to make sense of, heal, and unite dysfunctional and functional ego states, including specific therapies like the Structural Dissociation Model, Internal Family Systems, Life-Span Integration, the Developmental Needs Meeting Strategy, Imaginal Nurturing, and a few of the many general techniques for working with states in traumatized clients.

INTERNAL FAMILY SYSTEMS

Richard Schwartz developed IFS based on family systems theory. He sees ego states in the context of the entire system, realizing that for a part to change, the entire whole must transform. He believes that everyone has an undamaged, compassionate, confident, curious Self that must be accessed by and allowed to lead each person's system.

[IFS creates] access to the Self, and then working through the Self to heal parts of the mind . . . results in clients becoming able to live more fully in a state of self-leadership. Rather than dealing with a client whose Self is obscured and blended with parts, or dealing directly with a client's parts, the IFS therapist works as a partner to the client's Self, and the client's Self becomes the compassionate therapist or leader with the parts. (Twombly & Schwartz, 2008, p. 296)

In IFS, parts are conceptualized as whole personalities, with their own temperaments, ages, and talents. Parts carry troublesome burdens from traumatic events, which need to be dislodged from the systems. They often hold opposing feelings and functions, though some can ally with each other. The therapist's job is to facilitate the Self to create alliance, understanding, and respect between parts; "to help clients reach and maintain a state of self-leadership in which they can heal themselves" (Twombly & Schwartz, 2008, p. 298).

There are three kinds of parts: managers, exiles, and firefighters (Schwartz, 1995). Manager parts are protectors that work to keep their person safe and healthy and away from the feelings of the exiles. They can be inner critics, workaholics, or codependents who strive to keep needed people around. Note the similarity to SD's apparently normal parts. Exiles, like SD's emotional parts, often contain the experiences and feelings of and reactions to the trauma. Firefighters may frantically use substances, behavioral addictions (cutting, sex addiction), or other means to distract the Self's attention from exiles that are too present or too intense. "For any part to unburden, it needs to feel connected to and be fully witnessed by the Self in whatever way is necessary for that part to feel comprehensively known" (Twombly & Schwartz, 2008, p. 303).

IFS Steps to Healing

1. Accessing the Self by unblending from the parts. You know it's the Self by its compassion and curiosity toward the other parts.

2. Witnessing: Each part allows itself to trust the Self and expect the Self to understand its beliefs, burdens, and feelings.

3. Retrieval by the Self of the parts from the past that they think they live in. The Self finds the part and brings it to the present (a component of many kinds of ego state work).

4. Unburdening: The parts, when willing, unburden the feelings or beliefs they carry, up in the air, by fire, or any way that works in their imagination.

5. Parts replace the burdens with positive qualities. "What do you want to have where that burden or feeling used to live?" Often, it is peace, hope, energy, warmth, and possibility.

6. Integration and reconfiguration of the system: Unburdened parts may merge with other parts or get a new role in the system.

7. Checking for questions and concerns. At the end of an IFS session, the therapist asks the Self to check and see if there are any parts that have concerns or comments. Each concern and comment needs to be heard and addressed. (paraphrased from Twombly & Schwartz, 2008, pp. 300–301)

While it's not in the steps to healing, an important part of IFS is the Self of the therapist. Schwartz wants IFS therapists to be in their own Self as they work with clients. Dissociative clients can create massive countertransference in many good therapists. When therapists start out in their oldest, wisest Selves, they have a chance to stay grounded throughout the therapy. When therapists notice being pulled away from their Selves, it can be helpful information while doing any kind of therapy.

Discussion

IFS hits all the bases of good ego state therapy, from strengthening the Self through bringing the parts to the present and allowing all parts to connect with the here-and-now Self, to unburdening and clearing the trauma and cognitive distortions, to installing positive energy and affect, to checking each part at the end. It can work with simple trauma, small-t relational trauma, or extreme dissociation.

IFS Resources

Richard Schwartz, *Internal Family Systems Therapy* (Guilford, 1995). The bible.

The Center for Self Leadership, available at http://www.selfleader ship.org/. The Web site.

Joanne Twombly and Richard Schwartz, "The Integration of the Internal Family Systems Model and EMDR," in C. Forgash and M. Copeley (Eds.), *Healing the Heart of Trauma and Dissociation With EMDR and Ego State Therapy* (Springer, 2008).

LIFE SPAN INTEGRATION

LI is a systematic way of bringing "an exchange of energy and information between the minds of adult and child" states (LI Web site, http://www.lifespanintegration.com, accessed November 11, 2009). The inventor of LI, Peggy Pace (2007), has continued to develop and expand it since 2002. It's simple, clear, and ritualized. Here is how it goes:

1. Start with a childhood trauma. The adult part describes the event, the age of the child, the affect, and the bodily sensations that go with it.

2. The adult goes back in time to the child, introduces himself or

herself, and takes the child out of the situation to a safer place in that time.

3. The therapist coaches the adult to tell the child some appropriate positive cognitions, for example: "You're with me now." "You're safe." "It wasn't your fault." "You're a good girl."

4. The adult takes the child by the hand and takes her on a tour of the years, year by year, until the present. If the client's life was relatively benign, she can simply be coached to remember one event, good, bad, or neutral, for each year, as the therapist intones, "5 years old [pause], 6 years old, 7 years old," and so on, until the present year. If the client had an abuse-filled or desolate life, the therapist reads from a prepared list of good or benign events that occurred in each year. "Nice third grade teacher, winning the spelling bee in fourth grade, trip to Grandma's," and so on. With clients older than 40, you can start skipping years after 25, going every other year.

5. When they reach the present time, have the adult part orient the child part to the here and now, including the adult capabilities. "Show that child that you live in a safe place now. Show that child how you do so well at your job. [Specify.] Show that child your sweet spouse and all of the people who love you now. Show her how you take care of your outside children. How is that child now? Is she ready to blend with you?" If not yet, she can hang out, for now.

6. Then go back to the original trauma. "What do you feel in your body now when you think of that event?" Specify. If there is any feeling left, repeat steps 2 through 5, until the feeling disappears, the child is no longer in the picture, or the client says he or she is completely done.

Discussion

LI is a tremendously integrative therapy. You can often see clients looking more grown up with each pass through the years. The ritual of coming up through the years can contain affect and trauma and build affect tolerance as you touch on each year for a moment and move on. As you repeatedly go up through the ages, clients will report that more positive memories come through with each round. LI can completely clear many kinds of childhood trauma, including attachment trauma or neglect.

Basic LI causes flooding in some DID clients, and should be used with caution with that population. I've found it useful with primary and secondary dissociation (scattered trauma to personality disorders). Peggy Pace has developed a Part II workshop with techniques for dissociation.

LI Resources

Peggy Pace's life span integration Web site is available at http://www.lifespanintegration.com/, including her manual and workshop schedule.

THE DEVELOPMENTAL NEEDS MEETING STRATEGY

DNMS therapy, developed by Shirley Jean Schmidt, is a structured, complex ego state therapy that "borrows from ego state theory, inner-child therapy, self reparenting therapy, developmental psychology, attachment theory, and EMDR" (2009, p. 18).

DNMS labels existing dysfunctional ego states as either controlling or powerless reactive parts (which correspond to the IFS firefighters and exiles) or simple or oppressive maladaptive introjects (parts of role models that have been taken on by the child) or reactive mimics, parts of the self that mimic the beliefs and abusive behavior of the maladaptive introjects. Maladaptive reactive introjects are differentiated by whether they hold the beliefs of the role model (simple), hold the abusive behavior (oppressive), or whether they arose during or after a trauma.

DNMS therapy consists of identifying and strengthening the felt sense of healthy, attachable adult Selves who become the healing circle and bring maladaptive ego states to the circle to be cared for and healed. The healing circle consists of a nurturing adult self (NAS), a protective adult self (PAS), and a spiritual core self (SCS). DNMS therapists read a list of nurturing and protective skills and traits, while clients think of a time they have done or shown each skill. "Think of that familiar experience of being naturally, effortlessly, and appropriately nurturing or protective as I name each skill on the list" (Schmidt, 2009, p. 51). Therapists repeat the list, with bilateral stimulation, and then say, "Now bring these skills together into a single sense of self, your nurturing/protective adult self, and tell me when it's strengthened all the way." After clients identify and strengthen their NASs and PASs, they create a mental picture of each of them.

The SCS corresponds to the IFS Self and is associated with feelings of interconnectedness, completeness and wholeness, safety and invulnerability, effortless happiness, acceptance, loving-kindness, compassion, wisdom, and both timelessness and the present moment. "Some people call it the soul. Some believe it is a part of self that existed before life and after the body dies" (Schmidt, 2009, p. 53). Therapists read a meditation to connect clients to the SCS, including deep breathing, recalling of spiritual states, and creating a mental picture of the SCS.

The NAS, PAS, and SCS comprise the healing circle, which meets the unmet needs of every maladaptive part of the self. They unmask introjects and tend all other parts. The DNMS creates a powerful way to bring adult capacities to distressed child parts for healing and integration.

In the manual and the training there are dozens of specific interventions for each part of the self, conference room protocols, needs-meeting protocols, and very specific interventions for what to do when the very specific protocols won't work.

Discussion

DNMS is a step-by-step protocol for identifying both adaptive and maladaptive parts and bringing them together in very specific ways for healing and integration. Shirley Jean Schmidt does an excellent job of explaining and differentiating different kinds of parts, introjects, and resources and giving us specific ways to work with them. The healing circle meeting the needs of the child parts is a powerful and helpful intervention. The unmasking techniques for introjects are lovely.

The DNMS protocol has some problems. It can be too rigid for some clients and some therapists, so it shouldn't be the only tool in your therapy box. It's very complex and can be unwieldy, even though the interventions are solid. Many therapists use parts of the protocol, adapting it to the needs of specific clients. Shirley Jean Schmidt has been publicly called out by some of the luminaries in the dissociation field for failing to cite their contributions to her technique.

DNMS Resources

The DNMS Web site, from which you can buy the very good manual or find a training session, is at http://www.dnmsinstitute.com/.

IMAGINAL NURTURING

April Steele has created a simple, powerfully healing technique that is rooted in attachment theory and research and is the heart of her developing a secure self (DSS) approach. It's simple. In the preparation phase for trauma therapy, the therapist reads one of two scripts to the client and sends the client home with a CD of what she read. Both scripts are present-tense encounters between the adult self and a child self. One features an infant, shortly after birth ("I'm So Glad You're Here!"); the other, a toddler ("Adventuring Spirit"). The scripts stress sensory information for both parts: "Feel the child's warm and heavy body in your arms, as you look into his beautiful alert eyes and he feels your strong arms around him and looks into your protective, warm eyes." Adults and babies feel, see, hear, and smell each other. The positive affect goes intersubjectively back and forth. Adults affirm the babies' lovability and acceptability.

The toddler script has become part of my cure for passive-aggressive personalities and some forms of codependence. In it, the adult holds the toddler in a room with a shelf of toys. The adult and toddler see and feel each other, connect, and enjoy each other's company. After a while, the toddler looks around at the toys and is encouraged to go play with them. The adult admires the playing toddler, who looks back for security. When the toddler begins to feel less secure, he looks back at the adult, who welcomes the child back with open arms. They feel, see, and hear each other once more, and reaffirm the connection. Then do the going away, playing, and the happy return again. After several rounds of the toddler script, passive clients have felt implicit permission to explore and to reach out for what they want, without fear of loss of relationship.

All four scripts (two for men, two for women) give child selves a chance to be admired and enjoyed, to know that they matter, to feel secure in knowing that there is always an adult around to look after "the adult stuff," to be held, and to hear appropriate messages. Every IN session ends with the client bringing the child into his or her heart.

Clients check in with child parts daily and are taught specific ways to connect with child parts when feeling distressed. Clients reinforce the attachment lessons by listening to IN CDs during the week. All week long, adult parts learn attachment skills and child parts experience being attached to a good, constant object.

There are three major components of DSS:

1. The therapeutic relationship: in which the warm, attuned, and responsive therapist addresses attachment issues at an implicit as well as an explicit level and speaks to the young ego states as well as to the adult.

2. Imaginal nurturing: the scripts, in which the process, imagery, and nurturing encouraging messages are responsively tailored to the individual client.

3. Emotional skills: "Clients learn to respond to the younger parts of self when they are feeling distressed, which promotes the relationship [between adult and self] and addresses the feelings" (IN Web site, http://www.april-steele.ca/nurturing.php, accessed August 29, 2009).

Discussion

IN does not try to be a complete psychotherapy. Created as an adjunct to EMDR, it can be a useful addition to the preparation phase of any trauma therapy with attachment-disordered clients. It's simple, safe, integrative, and very nurturing. Not every client likes it ("Don't give me that inner child stuff!"), but I've never seen anyone harmed by it. I've been delighted to experience big tough guys crying with joy while imaging holding their baby selves. I've been excited to hear parents say that their attachment skills have improved since they started listening to the IN CDs. Mostly, I've been gratified to see my attachment-disordered clients become more able to soothe themselves, accept themselves, love themselves, and become more whole.

IN Resources

You can read more about IN, buy the useful manual and CDs, or find out about training at http://www.april-steele.ca/nurturing.php.

WORKING WITH PARTS

Here is a partial compendium of ways to organize, connect, and integrate parts from many kinds of ego state therapies. When I know who invented them, I let you know.

Going Inside

The therapist might say, "Go inside and find out what part or parts of you is radiating this terror. The 4-year-old? What is she telling you? What do you know that she needs to know? Can you tell her now?"

This technique assumes:

1. You are talking to an adult part.
2. The needed information is "inside."
3. The presenting adult is in charge of dealing with all other parts (Calof, 2000, personal communication).

Conference Room

Often used with DID and DDNOS clients, the conference room or dissociative table (Fraser, 2003) is an imaginal place for ego states to show themselves, speak their minds, resolve conflicts, share information, and be oriented to the present. Some conference rooms are part of safe or healing places (Chapter 5). I've found conference rooms also help people with secondary dissociation, especially clients with borderline personality disorder. Here's an example of setting up a Conference Room with a client with Borderline Personality Disorder:

Therapist: You know how we've been talking about your parts: the grown-up part, the scared clingy kid, the angry part, and the shut-down, depressed part. Let's give them a place to talk to each other. Can you go to your healing place now? . . . Are you there? Great. I want you to create a room in that house for all your parts to get together. It needs to be big enough for a conference table, comfortable chairs, and enough room for all parts. . . . Got it? Make sure it's comfortable for everyone. Some of those parts are pretty young. They may need booster chairs. Got it? Perfect. Let's bring in the parts. Who is here?

Client: Adult me, angry me, depressed me, and scared baby.

Therapist: Who sits at the head of the table?

Client: The adult is, but the angry one wants to.

Therapist: Can your adult chair the meeting and keep order and make sure all parts get air time and their needs met? [Setting the rules and putting the adult in charge.]

Client: Sounds okay.

Therapist: So, Ms. Adult, who needs to talk first?

Some therapists chair the meeting and speak directly to each part. I try to work through the apparently normal parts, when possible, keeping in mind that I'm dealing with a system, not just parts.

Talking Through

Talking through is communicating to a part or parts in order to reach other parts. With a DID client, you might talk to the conference room of parts that you know, to parts who aren't yet known, by you or by the client. Or you may simply tell one part to pass on information to another. This works especially well as a way to reach shy or recalcitrant parts.

- Can you tell that terrified little baby that she's safe now? That you're with her?
- Let all the parts you know and all the parts you don't know understand that they live in 2010, that it's safe here, and no one will abuse you here. Let all the parts you know and all the parts you don't know yet, know that it's time, time to relax, time to enjoy the feeling of safety and freedom that comes with being in 2010, far away from the abuse.
- All parts at the conference table and all parts not at the table can know that they're safe now, that it's 2010 and the abuser isn't here, that this room is a safe place to be.

GENERAL EGO STATE THERAPY RESOURCES

Helen Watkins and John Watkins, *Ego States: Theory and Therapy* (Norton, 1997). One of the first and the best.

G. Emmerson, *Ego State Therapy* (Crown House, 2003).

C. Forgash and M. Copeley, *Healing the Heart of Trauma and Dissociation With EMDR and Ego State Therapy* (Springer, 2008).

Sandra Paulsen, *Looking Through the Eyes of Trauma and Dissociation: An Illustrated Guide for EMDR Therapists and Clients* (Bainbridge Institute for Integrative Psychology, 2009). A good guide for general parts work, whether or not you do EMDR. Simple enough for clients to understand.

The International Society for the Study of Trauma and Dissociation Web site: http://www.isst-d.org/

CHAPTER TWENTY

Structural Dissociation: Phase-Oriented Treatment

Pierre Janet (1859–1947), who many think to be the originator of modern psychotherapy, noticed that dissociation involved divisions among "systems of ideas and functions that constitute personality" (Janet, 1907, p. 332). Janet and his followers described phase-oriented treatment, including phase 1, symptom reduction and stabilization; phase 2, treatment of traumatic memories; and phase 3, integration and rehabilitation "to raise the patient's integrative capacity to improve function and resolve structural dissociation and related maladaptive behaviors" (Steele et al., 2005). Van der Hart and colleagues (2006) base much of their three-phase structural dissociation (SD) treatment model on the work of Janet.

You can review Chapter 2, "Dissociation," to remind yourself about apparently normal parts (ANPs), emotional parts (EPs), and the SD description of dissociation.

Phase 1: Stabilization

In the stabilization phase, therapists help clients to get over fears of attaching to and possibly losing the therapist or the good regard of the therapist, then help clients overcome their avoidance of the traumatic material and their dissociated emotions and parts. Therapists work with clients to identify and organize the ANPs and EPs that especially avoid therapeutic connection and thoughts or experience of the trauma. Gradually, clients and therapists get to know the ANPs and EPs in the clients' system. Tell clients, "We all have parts that pertain to our different ages and functions. When we have big traumas or littler ones over a long period of time, the parts get more closed to each other and less collaborative. It's our job to get them working together and under your most grown-up conscious choiceful control."

Phase 1 clients will often test the therapy relationship, finding answers to these questions: "Is the therapist really here for me?" "Can she handle my distress?" "Does she think I'm crazy?" "If she finds out how awful/screwed up/unlovable I am, will she leave?" "Is she really going to make me deal with all this horrible stuff?" The therapist's job is to pass all of the tests, while teaching the client what therapy and a therapeutic relationship are. In so doing, the therapist begins to heal the attachment wounds that every dissociated client brings to therapy.

Phase 1 is the time to begin to address self-harm, suicidality, substance abuse, and any self-destructive or stuck-in-the-past reactive decision making. Help clients strengthen the capacities of their most functional ANPs with questions and statements such as these:

- What does your oldest, wisest self think you ought to do about that?

- Is that your oldest, wisest self talking, or is it an angry, scared, shut-down kid part?

- Think about a time when you were on your game at work, present, running on all cylinders. How does that feel inside? We're going to work to get you to hang out in that part of you more of the time. And we're going to find pathways back to that part of you, when you end up in old stuff.

Help clients learn to tolerate and think about uncomfortable feelings, anger, loneliness, fear and panic, and especially shame. "As you sit with that fear, notice what you want to do to get away from it, and then just notice it and notice that I'm here with you and you're here, not back being abused. It's an awful feeling, but you're hanging with it!" (Notice the use of exposure and cognitive coaching here.) Sometimes I paraphrase Stephen Gilligan (personal communication, 1995): "It's the job of life to bring every feeling that a human can possibly feel through every human being. And it's the job of every human to allow life to run those feelings through us unimpeded, without holding on too tightly to the ones we like, or trying to block the ones we don't." If you engage the strongest, healthiest ANP, nearly any emotion can be withstood. And if that ANP can phone friends, use containment imagery (see Chapter 4) find something soothing to do, and connect strongly with you, the client can begin to cope with EP intrusions constructively. Steele et al. said, "In positive terms, Phase 1 is dedicated toward raising the integrative capacity of the ANP(s) and dominant EPs to allow for more effective functioning in daily life. The patient must gradually develop empathy for and enhanced cooperation among all parts of the personality, without yet sharing traumatic materials" (2005, p. 21).

PHASE 2: TRAUMA WORK

Phase 2 is the trauma work. You start with the client's ambivalence about the perpetrator(s). Clients who were close to the perpetrator(s) develop insecure attachments to them: intense loyalty, no matter what. Insecure attachment leads to defensive shame: "I'm bad. The abuse was my fault, because I need my mom/dad to be good and sane and strong or I won't survive. So it has to be my fault. So I'm not worth anything, so I deserved it" (Steele et al., 2005; Knipe, 2009). Identify the EPs (and possibly the ANPs) who are desperately clinging to the perpetrators and the EPs and ANPs who either defend against (feeling rage, hatred, or avoidance) or are recuperating from the abuse of the perpetrators. Have all of them notice that they're safe in the here and now. "The therapist can 'talk to' and 'talk through'" these parts, encouraging them to "look and listen, feel and focus on the present, where no one can come to you in this room" (Steele et al., 2005, p. 26). Elicit the EPs' and ANPs' empathy for one another. Getting them on the same page and attached to each other is important for the trauma work. You want the EPs to begin looking toward their older, wiser ANPs for support, mindfulness, and guidance or you will be co-opted into ANP status and subject to many more emergency phone calls. Begin to go after the cognitive distortions in this part of the preparation stage.

Other preparation tasks include these:

1. Continual monitoring of the window of tolerance: noticing when hypoarousal or hyperarousal is triggered (see Chapters 3 and 10).

2. Getting a sense of the beginning and ends of the traumatizing events, if possible.

3. Planning for extended sessions and outside support for the clients (rides after trauma sessions, if needed).

4. Explaining the work to the client and collaborate to plan it according to the client's needs.

5. If needed, sorting out which parts will and won't participate in any given working through of a trauma event (ANP helpers, yes; EP parts from other abusive situations, no). You can ask uninvolved parts to take naps, go play elsewhere, or reside in the safe place in "sound-proof, feeling-proof rooms" (Twombly, 2005). Kathy Steele says, "Apart from content, the planning focuses on the question of which parts should initially participate (one or more of the parts keeping aspects of the traumatic memory and parts that can fulfill a helping role) such as offering courage, structure or comfort—during or directly after synthesis" (2005, p. 28).

6. After the clearing, it's easier to confront cognitive errors such as, "It was my fault." Some of these errors are embedded in dissociated EPs.

In synthesis, you guide the chosen EPs and ANPs (including all of them, if appropriate for your client) through sharing the traumatic memories. In SD, you start with the least threatening and gradually go for the worst and most avoided part of the trauma, using many possible methods. However you do it, you must keep your clients in the window of tolerance: aroused enough to feel and do the work, not shut down, not overwhelmed, and still always with one foot in the here and now. You can use exposure, EMDR, imaginal reexperiencing, somatic work, the energy psychologies, or simply have the ego states share the memories.

A polyfragmented DID client who was fond of *Star Trek* used the "Vulcan mind meld" between parts. All involved EPs and ANPs would gather in a circle, EPs interspersed between older, wiser, grown-up ANPs. Parts that were not involved would "go to the beach," her safe place. This polyfragmented woman had an EP that held each of the strong emotions, and others that held different parts of the ritual abuse she had suffered. Here's how the trauma processing went, in about an hour, after more than a year of preparation, with some of the most gruesome parts edited out:

Client: We're all in the talking place, hand in hand in hand in hand in hand in hand. BT [a protective EP, very active in the system] is between grown-up Brenda and Nurturer [both ANPs] and she's letting them feel her fear and defiance as the men come in the room. She shows them how she went to Mother Goose Land when they got too close. [We had used the talking place many times before we tried trauma processing.]

Therapist: Who was there in the room next?

Client: The limp baby who has the pain [a dorsal vagal EP]. She squeezes Adult Brenda and the Nurturing One's hands and they feel and see what happened to her. The Nurturing One is crying, but she's okay [empathy between parts].

Therapist: What happens next?

Client: More men and more men and pain and being limp and knowing that this is what I'm for.

Therapist: Can you stay with it and let the grown-up ones help with the pain?

Client: Yeah.

Therapist: You grown-up parts, can you let her know it's not her fault, that these people were crazy psychopaths?

Client: Of course.

Therapist: Is BT willing to connect with the limp baby and feel some of this?

Client: She might kill someone! And then they'll kill her.

Therapist: I think it happened about 40 years ago and none of those guys are in this room [a matter-of-fact reminder].

Client: Oh, right. Okay. Baby and BT are holding hands and melding. [BT's voice starts to cry and yell.] I couldn't stop them [sobs]. I want to kill them. [After a while calms down.] No wonder I went to Mother Goose Land! [Sighs.]

Therapist: BT, could you and Baby go get hugs from Adult Brenda and the Nurturing One?

Client: That would be good. We're doing it.

Therapist: And did they see and feel what happened?

Client: Yeah.

Therapist: And are you and Baby okay?

Client: Yeah.

Therapist: Adult Brenda and the Nurturer, how are you doing?

Client: Okay, but mad and really sad.

Therapist: Good, it's worth being mad and sad about. I wonder if there's another part, after the abuse part that's physically passed out [an almost comatose recuperative-state EP we've seen before]. Adult Brenda, can you find her inside?

Client: Got her.

Therapist: Can you do a mind meld with her and find out what she needs?

Client: She doesn't know, but I know. She needs a bath and clothes and a long sleep and lots of hugs. [ANP to the rescue.]

Therapist: Do the other kids need that too?

BT: We say yes! We're going to the hot springs on the beach!

Adult Brenda: The Nurturer and I are going, too. [Describes how they put bubbles in the hot springs, and then powdered and dressed the kids and put them in the safe cabin on the beach for long sleeps.]

Therapist: What's it like to know the whole story?

Client: It still makes me mad, but it makes me understand why I am how I am. Now I'm sad.

Therapist: Can you breathe with that feeling for a while?

Client: Yeah. [Drips tears for a while, then looks up.]

Anger, then grief, is a normal response to clearing. Don't skip it.

Therapist: What do y'all need now? ["Y'all" can be singular or plural and can be very useful with this population.]

Client: We're okay. The kids are tucked in the safe cabin. We're hungry.

Therapist: That's a great sign of life! We just did a huge piece of work. Let's have a follow-up call tomorrow, to see how it goes.

How about 9 A.M.? [Schedule follow-ups early in the processing
to check if new parts pop up or for general containment.]

Client: That works.

Phase 3: Integration and Rehabilitation

In phase 3, clients learn to come full-fledged into their normal life,
connecting with others, doing healthy risk taking, and changing from
their old patterns of activity. They learn how to stop generalizing lessons from the abuse back then to here and now reality. They set goals
to do and be what to them would be formerly inconceivable. They
work through the grief of what happened and how that affected their
lives. Steele et al. said, "Phase 3 often involves deeper and more involved work related to severe developmental neglect suffered by the
patient, since increasing attempts to live normal life often highlight
less obvious deficits related to action systems that were not developed
adaptively" (2005, p. 41).

While some integration can occur in phase 2, in phase 3 you'll usually see more spontaneous integration of dissociative states. There are
many ways, beyond the scope of this chapter, to support or create this
fusion. With simpler childhood trauma, your client may simply "hug
that child until it's inside," as in the first example. The DID client in
the second case used her Vulcan mind meld to share the contents of
the minds of various parts until they united. Early on, integration is
tenuous, prone to breaking down when the client is traumatized by
external events or the nearly inevitable occurrence of new traumatic
memories. It takes a long time for a severely dissociated client (DID or
DDNOS) to hang onto integration. Some DID people let go of the
trauma, but maintain some highly differentiated parts, despite high
levels of function.

In phase 3, you might see your clients learn to play with others and
to experience bliss. A 64-year-old client discovered the joy of social
dance. A 60-year-old learned to say no for the first time, and thus could
tolerate an expanded social life, knowing that she could have and keep
boundaries, even in relationships. Several phase 3 clients had good
connected sex, with no intrusive memories and the ability to stay in
their adult selves, for the first times in their lives, in their 50s or 60s.
Each move forward brought grief with it. "I've been missing this all my

life." "I was too screwed up to have this before." Help them be with their grief. It will clear, and often you'll see their gratitude for their current lives arise.

CLINICAL WRAP-UP

The SD model is an all-purpose lens through which to see traumatized, dissociated clients. For me, it's the gold standard for treatment of highly dissociated clients. It's complex for a reason, naming the entire range of dissociative phenomena and giving us ways to prepare and contain our clients through all the stages of therapy. It "plays well with others," dovetailing well with many other trauma therapies and going beyond many of them, helping complex clients to integrate their new, nontraumatized selves into their new, expanded lives.

STRUCTURAL DISSOCIATION RESOURCES

O. van der Hart, E. Nijenhuis, and K. Steele, *The Haunted Self: Structural Dissociation and the Treatment of Chronic Traumatization* (Norton, 2006). The SD bible. Some find the language difficult, but it's worth the slog. A great basis for understanding every kind of dissociation and how to treat it.

K. Steele, O. van der Hart, and E. Nijenhuis, "Phase-Oriented Treatment of Structural Dissociation in Complex Traumatization: Overcoming Trauma-Related Phobias," *Journal of Trauma and Dissociation,* 6(3) (Haworth Press). The essence of *The Haunted Self* boiled down to 43 pages. I found it free online at http://www.onnovdhart.nl/articles/phaseoriented.pdf

Onno van der Hart's Web site is a trove of resources. Check it out at http://www.onnovdhart.nl/articles/

The International Society for the Study of Trauma and Dissociation often features van der Hart, Nijenhuis, and Steele at their annual conferences (http://www.isst-d.org/).

CHAPTER TWENTY-ONE

Treatments for Borderline Personality Disorder

"I won't work with borderlines." "She's such a borderline!" "Please don't refer any more borderlines." Why do some psychotherapists say these things about people with borderline personality disorder (BPD)?

People with BPD are often intense and easily triggered into overwhelming states of rage, terror, clinging, hopelessness, and depression. They can idealize people or things one moment and hate them the next. They often see the world and people in black-and-white terms, either all good or all bad. They are driven by the fear of abandonment, often staying in terrible relationships. Many people with BPD injure themselves with cutting, substance abuse, eating disorders, or fighting. They often try to medicate their out-of-control feelings with substance abuse or behavioral addictions (e.g., compulsive sex, gambling, Internet games, shopping). Some are chronically suicidal. They often see themselves as victims of others, though from the outside they may look like the obvious aggressors.

These people can be adult, charming, and wise in their ANP states, then switch immediately into fight, flight, cling (unmyelinated vagal) states, or completely shut down (dorsal vagal states) when triggered. Because of their constant state switching, many don't have a firm and steady sense of identity and may be confused about their professional paths, their values, and simpler identity issues.

BPD sufferers have had poor attachment experiences. Many of them suffered early childhood sexual and physical abuse. Because of this, they didn't have a chance to grow the right brain resources that would allow them to regulate their affect (Schore, 1994; Siegel, 1999).

Their intensely reactive emotions become overwhelming, easily triggered states and identities. Some conjecture that people with BPD have a genetic component that is then exacerbated by attachment or trauma experiences, including not having their enormous feelings validated by others (Linehan, 1993; Chapman & Gratz, 2007).

BPD sufferers can be challenging to psychotherapists. They may start out idealizing their therapists, then knock them off the pedestal at the first real or imagined error or hesitation to validate. Some, while in soul-crushing distress, may call or e-mail many times a day. Many are "cutters," with stripes of scars on wrists or legs. Some are frequently hospitalized for suicidal ideation or behavior. Some may express hatred and rage at the therapist. Most therapists, being human, would prefer to be validated for their niceness, not vilified for their inadequacies.

Luckily, people with BPD can be helped by a variety of psychotherapy techniques, and we therapists can have a chance to self-validate for hanging in while our clients' horrible distress and sometimes distressing behavior are allayed and they become whole. The rest of this chapter describes therapies useful with BPD clients.

DIALECTICAL BEHAVIOR THERAPY

Marsha Linehan (1993), has brought together cognitive, mindfulness, attachment, and good therapy principles in her dialectical behavior therapy (DBT), a comprehensive treatment for people with BPD and other related problems. DBT has two components:

1. Individual therapy that addresses suicidal or self-injuring behaviors, "therapy interfering" behaviors, and attendance at the skill training group. Therapists are available by phone to give clients support to apply the skills they are learning to their daily lives and to facilitate the inevitable need for relationship repair. The therapeutic relationship is warm and supportive. DBT therapists are strongly encouraged (and in some programs, required) to be in case consultation to deal with transference or countertransference issues that arise, and to stick to the program.

2. Skills training group, a 2½-hour weekly group that teaches core mindfulness skills (the capacity to pay attention, nonjudgmen-

tally, to the present moment), interpersonal effectiveness skills (e.g., assertiveness), emotion modulation skills (for conscious state change), and distress tolerance skills (how to deal with the self when big feelings are triggered).

DBT has four stages of treatment, which are completed before clients move on to the next:

1. Pretreatment: assessment, information about the therapy, and eliciting a commitment to the process
2. Stage 1: reduction of behaviors that are suicidal, self-injuring, therapy-interfering, and quality of life–interfering and growing the skills to resolve these problems
3. Stage 2: dealing with PTSD with exposure and cognitive-behavioral techniques
4. Stage 3: growing self-esteem and meeting individual treatment goals

DBT therapists validate their clients' emotions and behavior as understandable in the context of the client's past and current circumstances. They try hard to systematically reinforce targeted adaptive behaviors and to avoid reinforcing maladaptive behaviors. For instance, a client who phones after self-injury may not call again for at least 24 hours after the matter is dealt with.

DBT Training

DBT training will give any therapist skills for helping BPD clients and many others. It teaches firm boundaries, a variety of skills, and a comprehensive way of seeing and treating BPD. There are several levels of training, including introductory, foundational, and advanced courses for both individuals and teams. Marsha Linehan founded Behavioral Tech, her training organization (available at http://www .behavioraltech.org).

DBT Books

Marsha Linehan, *Cognitive-Behavioral Treatment of Borderline Personality Disorder* (Guilford, 1993). The explanation.

Marsha Linehan, *Skills Training Manual for Treating Borderline Personality Disorder* (Guilford, 1993). The techniques.

Linda Dimeff and Kelly Koerner (Eds.), *Dialectical Behavior Therapy in Clinical Practice: Applications Across Disorders and Settings* (Guilford, 2007). A book about using DBT in different settings with depression, substance use, eating disorders, suicide, psychosis, assaultive behaviors, and more.

DBT Self-Help

Matthew McKay, Jeffrey C. Wood, and Jeffrey Brantley, *Dialectical Behavior Therapy Skills Workbook: Practical DBT Exercises for Learning Mindfulness, Interpersonal Effectiveness, Emotion Regulation and Distress Tolerance* (New Harbinger, 2007).

Scott Spradlin, *Don't Let Your Emotions Run Your Life: How Dialectical Behavior Therapy Can Put You in Control* (New Harbinger, 2003).

A Web site by and for DBT clients with a good overview and helpful lessons is http://www.dbtselfhelp.com

OTHER THERAPIES FOR BPD

Therapists who work with complex trauma may use parts of many modalities to help their complex clients.

Structural Dissociation

Many therapists, including me, see BPD as a specific kind of dissociation and treat it accordingly. The structural dissociation (SD) therapy model starts with a stabilization phase, when clients have the integrative capacity and stable parts to do it. Trauma work is next, and then the integration and rehabilitation phases. SD successfully rounds up, supports, and heals BPD clients' distressed and acting-out dissociative states. (You can see how the DBT phases overlap with SD phases, with different methodology.)

Ego State Therapies

Ego state work is helpful in all stages of treatment of BPD, including internal family systems, imaginal nurturing, and lifespan integration. I sometimes use the old transactional analysis parent/adult/child circles to explain particular ego states. I have seen several high-functioning people with borderline features declare, "Oh, I'm an adult, not a kid! I can take care of myself!" after a few sessions of lifespan integration. Others, including much more dysfunctional clients, listen to the imaginal nurturing CDs daily, becoming more able to self-soothe and gain a sense of themselves as nurturing adults with each imaginal nurturing session.

Psychodynamic Therapies

The psychodynamic concepts of containment, projection, and relationship repair are essential parts of every therapy with clients who have BPD. BPD clients have broken attachments and need warm, connected, patient, boundaried therapeutic relationships to create new healthy attachment capacity. A big part of the therapy is parsing out what happened between therapist and client that triggered a particular response in session.

EMDR and Related Therapies

EMDR can be quite useful, especially for resource installation in the initial stages of treatment, trauma clearing in the middle stages, and skill practicing in the later stages. As a stand-alone therapy for BPD, EMDR requires huge attention to the stabilization phase of therapy. Maureen Kitchur's (2005) strategic developmental model (SDM) gives a chronological order to processing and creates ways to use EMDR with attachment and early trauma targets. Katie O'Shea (2009) provides an early trauma protocol for use with EMDR.

Since Carole Lovell (2005) starting using EMDR resourcing in her DBT groups and EMDR trauma processing in adjunctive individual sessions, she found that group members' suicidal and self-injuring behaviors and psychiatric hospitalizations fell close to zero; the clients were less internally disrupted, and the healing of the entire group moved more quickly and happened more completely.

Somatic Therapies

Both sensorimotor psychotherapy and somatic transformation are whole therapies that can provide somatic resourcing, trauma work, and integrative work for BPD clients. Many therapists use somatic work in conjunction with other therapies. Sandra Paulsen and Ulrich Lanius (2009) integrate somatic and ego state interventions with EMDR.

Energy Psychology

Thought field therapy, emotional freedom technique (EFT), and other energy psychologies are not complete therapies for complex trauma, but they can help BPD clients self-manage affective states in early therapy stages and can help clear trauma in middle stages of treatment. Because clients can take them home and do them by themselves, these therapies can reduce self-injuring behavior, hospitalization, and emergency phone calls. These therapies quickly give out-of-control clients a sense of control over their emotions and subsequent actions, thus raising self-esteem and self-efficacy.

A TYPICAL BPD CASE USING MANY MODALITIES

Janis had a rotten childhood. When we did the SDM genogram, we found that her mother was alternatively angry or depressed, possibly also suffering from BPD. Her father was alcoholic and emotionally and physically abusive. She'd been sexually abused by her older brother and a neighbor. In her 32 years, Janis had had and lost many jobs, usually getting fired. She'd had eight volatile relationships, tried and failed to complete college several times, and had five psychotherapists, all of which were now described as "horrible." According to Janis, I was the new idealized "great therapist" who was going to save her. When I heard this, I immediately warned her that I was prone to mistakes but good at working out consequences of them. Would she agree to let me know when I did something that didn't work for her, and stay around to work it out? She would. (We referred back to this promise many times when I became "bad.")

First we tracked her personal and family history with the SDM, paying special attention to attachment relationships, trauma, and the few areas of good connections and high function.

Early in therapy, I explained the structural dissociation model and she identified dissociative states that felt familiar: fight, flight, cling, and shut down. We talked about the strengths of her apparently normal part (ANP) and how we would try to keep that part in executive control, or at least in the room. We discussed the polyvagal system and how reflexive it had been for her to switch from normal connectable states into total fight or shut down. These discussions gave her a context for her formerly unexplainable and shameful state switches. She began to use less self-shaming language as we went along.

We made a plan:

1. We would start with EFT and grounding and breathing lessons to help her deal with overwhelming feelings.

2. We met twice each week, for extra containment and to get a jump on feeling better, until we both agreed to one session. (For about the first year.)

3. She would listen to the infant-oriented imaginal nurturing CD three to seven times each week. When she had enough of it, she would switch to the toddler tape, three to seven times each week.

4. If she wanted to quit therapy, she had to come talk to me in person before she did and work on relationship repair. (Many people with BPD fire their old "bad" therapists to hire a new "good" one.)

5. After 3 months of therapy, when she could be more comfortable in her body, she would join a regular yoga class.

6. We would go after black-and-white thinking with the two-hand interweave. "In one hand, hold that the world is completely against you, nobody could ever like you, and it all has always sucked. In the other hand hold that maybe it's not all about you. Maybe some people (like me) have great affection for you, and maybe, once in a while, it hasn't completely sucked. Stay with both hands and tell me what happens" (Shapiro, 2005).

7. If she felt like cutting, dying, or hurting someone else, she'd do her EFT routine first and her grounding and breathing. If that didn't work, she'd call me. (This is why I have an answering service.) After we had a chance to do some ego state work, we added that she'd have her oldest-wisest adult comfort the distressed part before she could call. If she did cut herself, we had to deal with that before we went on with any other issues.

8. When we both felt that she was stabilized enough, we would use EMDR, EFT, and Lifespan Integration directly on trauma memories. (At 8 months, we began, with frequent forays back

to grounding, repairing the relationship, and talking about how to deal with her life.)

9. The last goal was to integrate her new wholeness into her life: mindful choice of work, good relationships, and ability to enjoy her leisure time without having to deal with "the black hole of horrible feelings."

10. She got to stay in therapy (providing she didn't physically hurt me or my property) until she was ready to leave (allaying her abandonment fears, deepening her commitment and demonstrating my commitment, and giving her a sense of control).

The first months were rocky. She had almost no tolerance for stress. When she felt slighted, frustrated, or lonely, she wanted to strike out, run, or hurt herself. As she learned to identify the states and to use her new self-soothing techniques, she gained a sense of power over herself. I lost my idealized status after about 2 months, and much of our time was spent on relationship repair.

At about 8 months, still meeting twice each week, she felt able to sufficiently self-soothe and "hang onto her adult self, no matter what" so that we could begin the trauma work. Using Kitchur's SDM, we started with a target of her as a little baby in her depressed, nonconnecting mother's arms. As we went through the EMDR protocol, cognitions, emotions, and physical sensations, she referred to her imaginal nurturing CD: "I can feel that lonely baby's hopelessness, but it's not as bad as it would have been without the CD." She was able to tolerate the processing and move through to the end. "I'm holding that 'baby me' now!" Other targets of specific traumas were more intense, but her relief in clearing them was palpable. "I'm done with that one!" As we cleared old targets, current issues arose: many were tied to abandonment or perceived abandonment, others to her loneliness, and that she'd driven away many friends with angry outbursts. When I planned a vacation, we spent several sessions on her feelings of betrayal and abandonment. EMDR and TFT directly on the feelings were helpful, as was having another therapist see her once each time I was gone and be available for phone calls.

We began to use a modified lifespan integration with various abandoned child parts, having her oldest-wisest adult go back in time to the child, and bringing her up through the years until the present, to be held and "hugged in" to the adult. As we rescued each part, Janis reported that she felt older. When we moved through the sexual abuse, her horrible shame began to lift. "It wasn't my fault." "They were bigger." "Maybe I'm not disgusting." Through the work, we paid attention to her stance.

Therapist: Janis, how does your body feel when you know you're not disgusting?

Client: Lighter, taller.

Therapist: Can you accentuate that?

Client: Oh, yeah! It's like I can really breathe. And I'm really here.

Therapist: Go with that!

We integrated somatic work into much of the other work. If Janis was feeling frustrated, or like running, or hunkering down, I'd have her track it in her body, and then gently and slowly do the movement that expressed it. To her surprise, the feeling would lift. As she did yoga outside the sessions and was able to pay attention to and express emotion, her affect tolerance continually rose.

At 2 years of therapy, she told me, "I can feel mad without having to do something mad. I can be sad and not have to cut. It's sort of cool." Her emotions were no longer always tied to dissociative state shifts. I let her know how excited I was by this development (though I'd noticed it for a while). She stopped feeling like cutting. She rarely felt hopeless and depressed. And we began to look forward.

For the last 6 months, Janis tried on new behaviors. In the session, we practiced assertiveness. (Why blow up when you can simply say no?) She was already getting along better at work and beginning to make some tentative new social contacts. I had her practice cruising for friends. When I met her she was both gun-shy about all men and terribly lonely. Now, she felt less desperate, but still lonely, and we had discussions about finding a suitable man. What made a good one? Who should she avoid? How could she keep her hungry, lonely inner kids from picking someone just like her parents? How could she let the wisest parts of her pick a man? A friend? A job?

At 30 months of therapy she had reasonable tolerance for her affect, had ways to manage it, was well attached to me, though she saw me as less than perfect (a huge step), and could tolerate thinking about her past. She was in contact with her parents, with limits. When she tearfully said good-bye, we acknowledged the tremendous work we had done, and that I was available for refreshers.

Janis came back for two brief rounds of therapy. When she started to date the man who would become her husband, some old bad patterns of shame and fear and pushing away arose. With EMDR, we targeted some old family-of-origin issues, then some related here-and-now issues with her sweetheart, and then some potential future issues. Six weeks later, she was done.

At the birth of her first child, Janis experienced some grief about her own infancy and some fears about her ability to parent. We used EFT with the grief and fear. Then Janis resurrected her old imaginal nurturing CDs. After a week of daily listens, Janis told me, "I have everything inside me, now, that will allow me to nurture this child." I haven't seen her since.

CLINICAL WRAP-UP

Doing therapy with clients with BPD can be hair-raising. Few therapists look forward to the initial months of suicidal ideation or attempts, the possibility of hospitalization, dealing with cutting, sometimes dangerous eating disorders, and phone calls. Many therapists love to see the terror and rage subside, the attachment deepen, the idealization and vilification fall away, and dissociated parts begin to unify to a whole person who can tolerate and connect with others and self. For many of us, with whatever tools we use to get there, the journey and the outcome are deeply rewarding.

BPD RESOURCES

Professional Books

J. G. Gunderson, *Borderline Personality Disorder: A Clinical Guide* (American Psychiatric Publishing, 2001).

Mary Zanarini, *Borderline Personality Disorder* (Informa Healthcare, 2005). Medically oriented and horribly expensive.

Self-Help

Alexander Chapman and Kim Gratz, *The Borderline Personality Disorder Survival Guide: Everything You Need to Know About Living With BPD* (New Harbinger, 2007).

Robert Friedel, *Borderline Personality Disorder Demystified: An Essential Guide for Understanding and Living With BPD* (Da Capo, 2004).

Books for Family Members of People With BPD

Paul Mason and Randi Kreger, *Stop Walking on Eggshells: Taking Your Life Back When Someone You Care About Has Borderline Personality Disorder* (New Harbinger, 1998).

Randi Kreger and James Paul Shirley, *The Stop Walking on Eggshells Workbook: Practical Strategies for Living With Someone Who Has Borderline Personality Disorder* (New Harbinger, 2002).

Both give useful information and practical limit-setting and containment information for family and friends of people with BPD.

Part V

SPECIAL CASES IN TRAUMA THERAPY

CHAPTER TWENTY-TWO

Military

This chapter is more about the issues you might run into with military personnel than about the actual therapy. Each branch of the military has its own culture. If you're going to work with military personnel or veterans, you need to learn about the military in general, the branch to which your client belongs, the conflict in which your client fought, and his or her particular personal experience. You also need to know everything about your military client that you would know about any client. Trauma is easier to clear in anyone who went in with good affect tolerance, good attachment, and a premilitary low-trauma life. PTSD and other dissociative symptoms are most likely to develop in military personnel who had early attachment disruptions and childhood trauma.

Many people who join the military are from intact families and join with a sense of pride, responsibility, and belonging to something greater than themselves. A subgroup of people join because they don't function well, emotionally or otherwise, on the outside. These people will sometimes have preexisting conditions such as mental illness, poor attachment, or childhood abuse that will exacerbate trauma symptoms in treatment. Do a complete intake with every client.

War Trauma

From Silver and Rogers (2001), *Light in the Heart of Darkness*, here are some things to assess for in military personnel:

1. Duration of the exposure "contributes to erosion of an individual's capacities and modification of her or his perceptions while enduring combat" (p. 13).

2. The likelihood of multiple traumas.

3. That the trauma is man-made "has an added impact on an individual's world view, understanding of relationships, and sense of what it is to be human" (p. 14).

4. The tendency of a survivor to be both perpetrator and victim.

   • Objective perpetrators have committed acts seen as wrongful.

   • Subjective perpetrators have done acts that may be culturally sanctioned but violate their own deeply held moral beliefs.

   • Address atonement in therapy, often including how to give back to the community now.

5. There's a conflicted duality of the survivor's role, powerful and powerless.

6. Witnessing what happens to others, over and over: survivor guilt.

   • "Why did I survive?"

   • "Am I living a good enough life to deserve this survival?"

   • "I don't deserve a good life."

ASSESSMENT

Combat Operational Stress Versus PTSD

I interviewed Trisha Pearce, the director of the Soldiers Project–Washington in October 2009. She said that nearly every active-duty military person in combat situations has combat operational stress (COS). COS looks like PTSD, but it isn't. It's a reaction to the bizarre place and the constant danger. Full-blown PTSD needs a strong precipitating event. Typically, COS goes away over several months, and PTSD doesn't. She says that early treatment of COS can often keep clients from developing full-blown PTSD. She says that explaining to clients about COS destigmatizes a trauma diagnosis.

Assessment Issues Particular to Military People

The following list of assessment issues comes from Trisha Pearce and me:

- Are you dealing with someone from a military family? Is there transgenerational trauma? Was it passed down to your client?
- Assess clients for suicide. Do they still have weapons? If they're doing trauma work, will they be safe?
- Higher suicide risk: if his buddy got killed or if he is the only unwounded person in the unit, there may be survivor guilt.
- Is your client a National Guard or Reserve person who became a frontline defender? He may not have had as much preparation or expectation as an Army GI or Marine that he would be in active combat, so may have more risk for PTSD.
- It's not the job description, but what happened to them: People in Kuwait in the Gulf War may have been supposedly safe behind the lines, but may have seen vehicles with blood and guts on them and been traumatized. Medical personnel in Germany see every badly wounded person from Iraq and have trauma from what they see (Pearce, personal communication, October 2009). Drivers in Iraq, often women, frequently see combat.
- Was your client a minority in his or her squad? From another branch of the military? Different gender? Different in any other way? Was she or he part of the group or a pariah?
- Was the commanding officer supportive, stern, or abusive? Was your client singled out for abuse of any kind?
- Was there a sexual assault or sexual harassment? (This can happen to men or women.)
- Did the person suffer an explosion, car accident, or blow to the head that caused a traumatic brain injury (TBI)? Explosive shockwaves go straight through people and can injure organs, including the brain. TBI symptoms include the following:
  1. Out-of-control affect
  2. Confusion
  3. Lost time
  4. Headaches

5. Short-term memory deficits
6. Cognitive deficits that didn't exist before
7. Social deficits, no science of mind, no ability to read others
8. Can mimic the effects of dissociation

TREATMENT ISSUES

Therapist's Attitude

If you don't respect military people or have a strong opinion about any particular war or can't understand why an obviously traumatized client wants to go back to his or her unit, either keep it to yourself or go work with another client population. Trisha Pearce told me, "Keep your own politics out of it. Go with where your patient is."

Some clinicians become horribly traumatized from the material that military people bring back from the war zones. From the beginning, get good consultation support. Second, make sure you've done your own work. If it's still too much, let someone else do the work. You don't want your reactions to constrain your clients from sharing their experiences. And many of these folks will do anything to protect you.

Military Attitudes Toward PTSD

While top-down attitudes toward PTSD have changed in recent years, and new recruits are now taught to monitor the signs of distress and PTSD in themselves and others, there is still widespread disapproval of "not handling it." Commanders and squad leaders may not release their people for scheduled appointments, may discriminate against personnel who show signs of stress, and may not believe in the diagnosis. Soldiers, marines, and sailors are supposed to be tough. Having PTSD isn't being tough. Add societal attitudes about psychological problems to the mix, and you will have clients who are reluctant to come in and to face a PTSD diagnosis. Some avoid therapy or see off-base therapists, in order not to jeopardize their careers.

Veterans

Veterans may come to you for any kind of problem. Many don't have PTSD. Many do. Do a thorough intake, including their military service. I've worked with people who came in for current relationship issues, 30 years after deployment in Vietnam, for whom the underlying history of childhood neglect or abuse was the main driver of current dysfunction. After we cleared the early trauma, each said, "By the way, could we work on this thing that happened in Nam?" and we refocused the therapy. Other vets may come to therapy clearly traumatized by combat events, while missing the camaraderie and sense of purpose that they had in the military.

Active Duty

If you're working with active-duty people, approach the trauma differently. They want to go back. They want containment of the anxiety and trauma. Trisha Pearce commented, "It's not our job to keep them from going back." Do the fastest trauma work you can and give them tools for the road. Many active-duty people and some veterans can't explain the exact trauma, because it's classified. Find a way around it, with ritualized interventions. I've used EMDR, TFT, and stress inoculation for active-duty clients. As they say, "It gets 'er done."

Head Injury

Head-injured clients might need extra help to get to the sessions. Most have memory issues. Call them before appointments, or if they miss appointments, call to reschedule. Do short sessions, more frequently. Prepare to do a lot of problem solving. PTSD can co-occur with TBI. You have to treat both. Steven Silver (2009) says that EMDR can often clear the trauma of clients with TBI, since it works quickly and doesn't focus on the cognitive. I've found that EMDR and TFT can help organize clients who have head injuries, improving memory and clearing the trauma.

Sexual Assault

For both men and women, the worst part of sexual assault is often that the assailants are the people who are supposed to be protecting them. Due to pressure and attention from the top brass on down, and the higher number of women in the service, the number of sexual assaults in the Iraqi and Afghanistan wars is much less than in other wars. It still happens. And it's vastly underreported. You need to clear both the distress of the assault and the betrayal and helplessness of it (especially if the perpetrator was a commanding officer).

Adaptive Versus Pathological Dissociation

Dissociation can be adaptive. Combat personnel are trained to dissociate from their own fear and to focus on their mission. Don't confuse adaptive dissociation, a hyperfocus on a task, with pathology. Of course, a client with poor attachment, an early abuse history, and a preexisting tendency to dissociate may present extreme dissociation after the trauma of combat. As his or her therapist, you need to address their training versus unhelpful traumatic dissociation in the therapy.

In current conflicts, military people may be participating in battle one moment and on the phone or e-mail in the next. The "pilots" of drone planes may be sitting in the United States and witnessing people being killed on the drone cameras for a 12-hour shift, then picking up the kids and going home. This new ability to shift from one reality to another may promote more dissociation in some people.

Guilt, Shame, and Atonement

Military people are charged by our society to protect us at any cost. Sometimes they destroy property. Sometimes they scare people. Sometimes they injure and kill people. Sometimes they make mistakes. And sometimes they are unable to save or protect their fellow combatants. All of the above can go against the values of the most gung-ho soldier. Help your clients deal directly with the clash of ethics and the ensuing guilt. Point out the clash. Silver and Rogers (2002) wrote:

1. Help them examine the context of their traumatic, guilt-inducing event(s):

    a. It was war.

    b. I was ordered to _____.

    c. I didn't know _____.

    d. This was the circumstance: _____.

    e. This was my internal state, emotions, level of fatigue: _____ _____.

    f. I truly could/could not have done something different: _____ _____.

    g. I am/am not forgivable:_____.

2. If whatever trauma therapy you use does not completely clear

the guilt, shame, and moral distress of your client's actions or limitations, cocreate an atonement task. The three principles of tasks of atonement are:

a. Sacrifice. It should place a demand on the client that would not otherwise be there. [It should be hard enough that the person feels they're really doing something.]
b. Look outward. It should be something that benefits others.
c. Make use of client abilities. It should have something the client can realistically do, or rapidly obtain the skills to do. (2002, p. 193)

Atonement tasks often involve volunteering and might correspond, in a reparative way, to the action that created the guilt: volunteering with children, if a child was involved; helping at a vets' center, if it was about the failure to save a fellow soldier; and so on. I know Vietnam veterans who are still volunteering. One says, "This is how I know that I'm a good person."

CLINICAL WRAP-UP

Many of us enjoy working with military people for their courage, their unfailing courtesy, and their commitment to doing what they need to do. Society puts heavy burdens on its soldiers. To work with them, you need to understand their culture, their ethics, their burdens, and their underlying humanity. Some therapists are afraid to work with the life and death issues that military people face. Some are afraid that they won't relate to military people. There are thousands of traumatized military personnel returning from Iraq and Afghanistan at this writing. I hope many of you will pursue work with this underserved population. They need you.

RESOURCES

TBI

BrainInjury.com (http://www.braininjury.com): General information about traumatic brain injury (though run by lawyers).

Betty Clooney Foundation, About Traumatic Brain Injury (http://www.bcftbi.org/aboutSoldiers.asp): Soldiers with TBI, including referral and treatment information.

General Information

Healing Combat Trauma Web site (http://www.healingcombattrauma.com/).

U.S. Department of Veterans Affairs, National Center for PTSD (http://www.ptsd.va.gov/professional/index.asp).

U.S. Department of Veterans Affairs (http://www.va.gov): Get your veterans to utilize the VA. It's got good health care and many, many helpful programs.

Volunteering

Give an Hour (http://www.giveanhour.org): A national network of volunteer therapists. You do an hour of therapy per week, and your veteran or active-duty client donates an hour of his or her time to a good cause.

The Soldiers Project (http://www.thesoldiersproject.org) has sites all over the country. You volunteer with a veteran or an active-duty person until that person is done with therapy. You must be a licensed therapist and have some training on working with military personnel, which they often provide.

Paid Work

Military One Source (http://www.ceridianprovidersolutions.com).

Military Family Life Consulting Program (http://www.mhn.com/provider/start.do).

TRICARE, 1-877-TRICARE (877-2273). In some regions, Tricare doesn't accept EMDR.

Books

Ilona Meagher and Robert Roerich, *Moving a Nation to Care: PTSD and America's Returning Troops* (Ig Publishing, 2007). A general information book that defines the problem.

Bret Moore and Arthur Jongsma, *The Veterans and Active Duty Military Psychotherapy Treatment Planner* (Wiley, 2009). Forms and behavioral lists for many issues.

Daryl Paulson and Stanley Krippner, *Haunted by Combat: Understanding PTSD in War Veterans, Including Women, Reservists and Those Coming Back From Iraq* (Praeger, 2007).

Steven Silver and Susan Rogers, *Light in the Heart of Darkness: EMDR and the Treatment of War and Terrorism Survivors* (Norton, 2002).

Sebastian Junger's *War* (Twelve, 2010) examines the cohesion and courage in a group of army soldiers in Afghanistan.

Movie

The 2006 PBS documentary *The Carrier* is a 10-episode show about the functions and especially the people aboard the USS *Nimitz*, during its 2005 deployment to the Gulf. I've never seen a better depiction of military culture.

CHAPTER TWENTY-THREE

Grief and
Traumatic Grief

Grief is often traumatic, but does not always cause PTSD or other diagnosable conditions. It is a natural part of recovery from trauma, when clients grieve that the event or situation happened and how it impacted their lives. Traumatic stress exacerbates the grieving process, which often can't complete until the trauma is cleared.

SIMPLE GRIEF

Whether my clients have had a bad breakup, a death of someone close, or have lost their jobs, I explain grief to them. This is an excerpt from a letter to a friend who lost an adult child to a drug overdose. It covers all the bases that I walk through with my clients:

> It's the day after the funeral. You've done the ritual things. What now? The pattern goes like this: Numb, during which you can plan a funeral and sort of function, then Anger (which can hold Blame, of your kid, your self, the Universe, God, Fate, and anyone else, including your beloved). Anger can come out at the guy who cuts you off in traffic, the slow clerk, the dog, or anyone. Tell yourself it's grief, and don't hit anyone. Sadness is next, and it can cut to Hopelessness and Despair and Depression pretty easily. You need to keep remembering that these are inevitable feelings, not definitions of either yourself or reality. You'll cycle through all these feelings over and over, as reality keeps punching you, and you, somehow, keep knowing anew that your son is gone. After much longer

than you may think reasonable, you'll start to integrate the reality a little at a time. You'll be able to remember your son more clearly from happier times. You'll smile more. Then you'll see some kid who looks just like him, and the wave will knock you down again. After a while the waves get smaller and you get bigger, encompassing more of your life, even liking it again. My mother and other mothers who lost kids say you never get over it, but it gets easier. My own experience of grief is that the acute phase ends after far too long and then you simply miss the person, without feeling punched in the stomach or knocked over, just missing. Here are the four rules for grief that I came up with for my clients:

1. Grief always hurts far more than you think it should.
2. It always lasts far longer than you think it should.
3. As a process, grief sucks, and has nothing to recommend it. It makes you feel tired, angry, sad, and hopeless.
4. Slowly, it moves through and you end up merely missing, not pining, for the lost one.

TRAUMATIC GRIEF

Traumatic grief is different. It's a dissociative experience. It looks like PTSD. It can have flashbacks or obsessional thoughts and states about or from the following:

1. The phone call or event in which your client found out about the death.

2. The event that caused the death.

3. Pathological guilt and shame. (All parents think they should have prevented harm to their child; these states can exist in any parent.)

4. A changed sense of identity. (Who am I without that person?)

5. Traumatic events from the illness or medical interventions or the death itself.

6. The place where the person died or where he or she lived.

7. The miscarriage.

8. Activities that used to involve the person.

Trauma is cumulative. So is grief. Clients with poor attachment, dissociative states, or former traumatic loss, might have enormous trauma reactions from relatively small current losses.

So what do you do?

1. Use your relationship to warmly contain and validate what your client is going through.

2. Explain the grief process (see above) and that the client has a trauma reaction that may be blocking it. Explain how you understand that in these particular circumstances.

3. Use your fastest and best trauma therapies to move the trauma part.

CASE EXAMPLE: HELPLESSNESS AT A SPOUSE'S DEATHBED

An old-time client lost his wife to a horribly wasting cancer. A few weeks before she died, the regular, pain-aware physician left town and the new doctor didn't provide adequate medication. Three weeks after the death, the husband came in saying, "All I can remember is her writhing in pain and calling out to me. I couldn't do anything. It's all I see. I know I should have been able to do something." I explained the reenactment protocol to him and about the superhuman powers he should imagine.

Therapist: When you think about Susan writhing in pain, where do you feel it in your body?

Client: My stomach.

Therapist: Let your power arise from that sensation in your stomach.

He imagined a beam coming out of his stomach that passed through his wife, taking all the pain with it. When her pain was gone, he imagined the beam changing to a soothing, enveloping cloud that helped her sleep. At that point he started laughing and said, "It's okay, now. She's dead, and she'll never hurt again." The laughter changed abruptly to tears. "But she's gone now. I'll never see her again. [Sobbing.] For the first time in 3 weeks, I know that she's gone! But this grief is different than that horrible image of her in pain. That's completely gone. But this is horrible, too!"

I saw him several more times for normal grief therapy, explaining the grief process, encouraging him to join a widowers' group and to use his other social supports, and teaching him some thought field therapy tapping that he could use at home to keep the grief moving through. We used EMDR on some other specifically traumatic events: the day of the diagnosis, his wife's emaciated body, the day they realized that she would die, some of the medical procedures, and the day of the death. When he left therapy, he told me, "I'm still grieving, but it's the normal stuff. I can deal with it now and I have good support outside."

RESOURCES

Books About Grief

William Worden, *Grief Counseling and Grief Therapy: A Handbook for the Mental Health Practitioner* (Springer, 2009, updated 4th edition).

Judith Cohen, Anthony Mannarino, and Esther Deblinger, *Treating Trauma and Traumatic Grief in Children and Adolescents* (Guilford, 2006). A CBT-based treatment book.

Karen Katafiasz, *Grief Therapy* (Elf Self Help, 1995). A lovely, brief self-help book.

Peter McWilliams, Harold Bloomfield and Melba Colgrove, *How to Survive the Loss of a Love* (Prelude Press, 1993). A classic.

CHAPTER TWENTY-FOUR

Sexual Assault and Sexual Abuse

We humans think we should be able to control our own bodies. When we can't control what happens to us and what happens inside of us, we almost always blame ourselves. Every rape survivor I've met has felt shame about the event, saying, no matter what the circumstance, "I should have been able to stop it." Other issues often include these:

1. The feeling of being forever tainted or ruined (sometimes culturally reinforced).

2. Pervasive fear, depending on the circumstances, of going out, of being in the dark, of sleeping, of sexual situations, of men, of touch.

3. Intensely visceral flashbacks in whatever body part took the brunt of the assault.

4. Changed feelings toward the body or body parts: "It betrayed me." "It's ugly now." "I hate my body." "It's not mine anymore." "It's disgusting." "I'm disgusting."

5. Male survivors often have questions about their sexuality and gender. "Does this make me gay?" "I feel like I'm not a man anymore." They often feel isolated, and even more shame, for not being able to protect themselves, like "real men" could.

6. More shame and confusion if their bodies responded sexually to the assault.

When people are assaulted by loved ones or trusted adults, another set of issues arises:

1. "I can't trust anyone anymore."

2. "What's the matter with me for loving/having loved that person?"

3. Or the unconscious belief, "Since I need to see him as good, I must be the bad one that made him do this thing to me. Therefore I am evil."

When people are sexually abused as small children, nearly always by adults or older children in positions of trust, they often believe, "Not only did I cause this to happen, by my badness, but this [sex and being abused] is what I'm for." Many prostitutes and some people with sexual addictions, when in therapy, find this belief underlying their life choices.

Early sexual and physical abuse, coupled with poor attachment experiences, are direct routes to dissociation. Few children stay present and whole while being raped by an adult. When the abuse is pervasive, the dissociation deepens, and the child becomes socially, behaviorally, and emotionally disrupted. Childhood sexual abuse is often a factor in creating DESNOS, borderline personality disorder, DDNOS, and DID.

When working with adult-onset rape survivors, clinicians must deal directly with the visceral experiences, shame and other emotions, disrupted trust, and distorted cognitions. When working with people who were sexually abused as children, clinicians must use therapies that can deal directly with child states and deep disruptions of self-cohesion and self-acceptance. In both cases, healed clients will be the following:

1. Free of flashbacks

2. Comfortable in their bodies

3. Safe in their lives

4. Able to rationally assign responsibility for the assault

5. Shame free

6. Able to enjoy a healthy sexual life

7. Able see themselves as worthwhile and untainted

My favorite phone message, ever, was from a woman who had been molested several times as a child. She had had 2 years of good cognitive behavior therapy before seeing me, which had caused most of the spontaneous flashbacks and thoughts of feeling dirty to abate. However, any sexual contact with her extremely sweet husband brought the flashbacks and frozen state back into her. After an intake and three EMDR sessions, she called me and said, "Robin, after 12 years of marriage, I just had the first sex of my life without feeling my grandfather in the room. It was wonderful. Thank you!" In two more EMDR sessions, she was completely free.

RESOURCES

Books about Incest

Christine Courtois, *Healing the Incest Wound: Adult Survivors in Therapy* (Norton, 2010, 2nd edition). A classic.

Christine Courtois, *Recollections of Sexual Abuse: Treatment Principles and Guidelines* (Norton, 2002).

Self Help

Aphrodite Matsakis, *The Rape Recovery Handbook: Step-by-Step Help for Survivors of Sexual Assault* (New Harbinger, 2003).

Ellen Bass and Laura Davis, *The Courage to Heal: A Guide for Women Survivors of Child Sexual Abuse, 20th Anniversary Edition* (Harper, 2008, 4th edition).

CHAPTER TWENTY-FIVE

Relational Trauma

Relational trauma can occur outside of the family and may not occur with people to whom one is attached. Here are some examples. All make good targets for trauma therapy.

1. Being the only black, Asian, Jewish (etc.), foreign, poor, rich, really smart, disabled, or different kind of person in a homogeneous classroom, military unit, office, or social situation.

2. Being singled out for any of the above by a teacher or other powerful figure.

3. Not fitting into one's upper-class milieu by being too fat or too expressive.

4. Not fitting into one's working-class milieu by being too smart or too refined.

5. Being bullied, at any age.

6. Being humiliated or shamed in front of other people.

7. Being humiliated or shamed by just one person.

8. Domestic violence.

9. Being rejected by a love object.

10. Grief.

11. Betrayal.

12. Embarrassment.

13. Demotion or unemployment.

14. Torture.

15. Having to keep a secret that sets you apart.

16. Having one's needs ignored, at any age.

All of these situations can create trauma. Any of them, chronically experienced, can root deeply into human neurology, creating a distorted view of the self ("I'm not worth caring about"; "I'm bad"; "Anything I try to do is futile"), depression, and psychological defenses against those experiences and people who might re-create them.

Any good trauma therapy may be effective with relational trauma, especially if it has a cognitive component. Go after the traumatic events and the concurrent beliefs about the self. Use your warm, connected therapeutic relationship to provide a counter to the destructive relationship of the past. It will be hard for your clients to buy into the idea that they don't matter, when they can feel that they matter to you.

Part VI

SELF-CARE

CHAPTER TWENTY-SIX

Self-Care for Trauma Therapists

As trauma therapists, we are privileged to watch our clients' trauma fade from terrible, here-and-now experiences to mere memories, their dissociation shift to integrated presence, and their pain disappear. We are also privy to the gut-wrenching details of rape, accidents, war, and story after story of child abuse, domestic violence, and horrible neglect. The more terrible the abuse and the more dissociated the clients, the more they project the actual emotions of their trauma into us. Some therapists become grim. Some avoid complex trauma clients. Some help their clients avoid expressing affect in the sessions. Some burn out and leave the profession. Some become vicariously traumatized and begin to feel avoidant about particular clients, or work in general. Here are some ways to keep yourself whole while doing this important work.

1. Do your own work. If you're not able to tolerate your own history and your current affect, you won't be able to tolerate the despair, rage, shame, and grief that move through many trauma survivors.

2. Learn mindfulness. Meditate or do yoga, qigong, or breathing exercises. It will help you "stay in the chair" while witnessing whatever is there to see. Learn to breathe and ground yourself while being with anything.

3. Know yourself. If you start a session in a state of equilibrium, and you start feeling rage or exhaustion in the session, guess that it may be the client's rage or dissociation. You may then

say, "What are you feeling right now? There's something in the room." The client is likely to say, "Oh, I'm angry. I guess it's about X." Or, "Oh, I was just spacing out." When you know where you are, you'll know when you are being drawn into someone else's experience and use it for their benefit.

4. Know the signs of burnout and vicarious traumatization:

   • You aren't excited to go to work.

   • You talk only about work and have no other interests.

   • You treat everyone on earth like a client.

   • You dream about clients, especially bad dreams.

   • You're angry at clients for being the way they are.

   • You feel shame for your human limitations.

   • You have vicarious trauma reactions: flashbacks, anxiety, depression, or avoidance around client material.

   • You want to drink, gamble, or otherwise dissociate after work.

5. Get support.

   • Join a supportive consultation group. (Not just about the technique, but about you, too. And no shaming allowed.)

   • Get individual consultation for the most troubling cases. As a consultant, I'm going step by step with a few consultees with their most fragile, barely tractable cases. It's good for the therapists and good for the clients.

   • Do your own work. Hire a good trauma therapist who can help you clear your vicarious trauma. If you have your own trauma history, you must deal with it, before your clients trigger your own unhealed wounds.

6. Increase your therapeutic arsenal. If what you're doing isn't working, find something else that does. Become a constant learner. The more lenses through which you can see your clients, the more interest and efficacy you'll have. The more effective you are, the less likely you are to burn out.

7. Develop other interests that have nothing to do with therapy. Make sure some of them involve unmitigated joy.

8. Do things that bring you into your body: run, stretch, work out, dance, do yoga.

9. If you have any control over your schedule and case load, limit

the number of the most complex, dissociated, abused, unstable clients. And don't see them all on one day.

10. You will probably learn your tolerance the way most of us do, by exceeding it. Once you know, keep your own boundaries. Follow the Platinum Rule: "Fill your own cup first; give away only what's left over." Another rule: "To thine own self be nice." Trauma is compelling, but don't let it run your entire life.

11. Watch out for grandiosity. You can't fix everything. Know your limits.

12. Know what's realistic. In the consultation group that I attend, all of us work with complex dissociated clients. It's helpful to see other people's clients inch forward when we all want ours to leap forward.

13. If you have a spiritual practice, use it to support your work. Ask whatever higher power you have for help when stuck.

This chapter was first published as a blog entry (at http://www .traumatherapy.typepad.com).

RESOURCES

Laurie Anne Pearlman and Karen W. Saakvitne, *Trauma and the Therapist: Countertransference and Vicarious Traumatization in Psychotherapy With Incest Survivors* (Norton, 1995). Written from a psychoanalytic perspective, it covers many bases.

Appendix of Trauma-Related Diagnoses

DSM Acute Stress Diagnosis[1]

A. The person has been exposed to a traumatic event in which both of the following were present:

   (1) the person experienced, witnessed, or was confronted with an event or events that involved actual or threatened death or serious injury, or a threat to the physical integrity of self or others

   (2) the person's response involved intense fear, helplessness, or horror

B. Either while experiencing or after experiencing the distressing event, the individual has three (or more) of the following dissociative symptoms:

   (1) a subjective sense of numbing, detachment, or absence of emotional responsiveness

   (2) a reduction in awareness of his or her surroundings (e.g., "being in a daze")

   (3) derealization

   (4) depersonalization

   (5) dissociative amnesia (i.e., inability to recall an important aspect of the trauma)

C. The traumatic event is persistently reexperienced in at least one of the following ways: recurrent images, thoughts, dreams, illu-

---

1. Reprinted with permission from the American Psychiatric Association (2000). *Diagnostic and Statistical Manual of Mental Disorders: DSM-IV-TR. 4th Edition.*

sions, flashback episodes, or a sense of reliving the experience; or distress on exposure to reminders of the traumatic event.

D. Marked avoidance of stimuli that arouse recollections of the trauma (e.g., thoughts, feelings, conversations, activities, places, people).

E. Marked symptoms of anxiety or increased arousal (e.g., difficulty sleeping, irritability, poor concentration, hypervigilance, exaggerated startle response, motor restlessness).

F. The disturbance causes clinically significant distress or impairment in social, occupational, or other important areas of functioning or impairs the individual's ability to pursue some necessary task, such as obtaining necessary assistance or mobilizing personal resources by telling family members about the traumatic experience.

G. The disturbance lasts for a minimum of 2 days and a maximum of 4 weeks and occurs within 4 weeks of the traumatic event.

PTSD[1]

DSM Definition of PTSD According to the *Diagnostic and Statistical Manual of Mental Disorders* (*DSM-IV*), post-traumatic stress disorder (PTSD) happens when:

A. a person is exposed to a traumatic event which is life threatening to themselves or others and experienced intense fear, helplessness, or horror.

B. The traumatic event is persistently reexperienced in one (or more) of the following ways:

(1) recurrent and intrusive distressing recollections of the event, including images, thoughts, or perceptions. Note: In young children, repetitive play may occur in which themes or aspects of the trauma are expressed.

(2) recurrent distressing dreams of the event. Note: In children, there may be frightening dreams without recognizable content.

---

1. Reprinted with permission from the American Psychiatric Association (2000). *Diagnostic and Statistical Manual of Mental Disorders: DSM-IV-TR. 4th Edition.*

(3) acting or feeling as if the traumatic event were recurring (includes a sense of reliving the experience, illusions, hallucinations, and dissociative flashback episodes, including those that occur upon awakening or when intoxicated). Note: In young children, trauma-specific reenactment may occur.

(4) intense psychological distress at exposure to internal or external cues that symbolize or resemble an aspect of the traumatic event.

(5) physiological reactivity on exposure to internal or external cues that symbolize or resemble an aspect of the traumatic event.

C. Persistent avoidance of stimuli associated with the trauma and numbing of general responsiveness (not present before the trauma), as indicated by three (or more) of the following:

(1) efforts to avoid thoughts, feelings, or conversations associated with the trauma

(2) efforts to avoid activities, places, or people that arouse recollections of the trauma

(3) inability to recall an important aspect of the trauma

(4) markedly diminished interest or participation in significant activities

(5) feeling of detachment or estrangement from others

(6) restricted range of affect (e.g., unable to have loving feelings)

(7) sense of a foreshortened future (e.g., does not expect to have a career, marriage, children, or a normal life span)

D. Persistent symptoms of increased arousal (not present before the trauma), as indicated by two (or more) of the following:

(1) difficulty falling or staying asleep

(2) irritability or outbursts of anger

(3) difficulty concentrating

(4) hypervigilance

(5) exaggerated startle response

E. Duration of the disturbance (symptoms in Criteria B, C, and D) is more than one month.

F. The disturbance causes clinically significant distress or impairment in social, occupational, or other important areas of functioning. (American Psychiatric Association, 2000, pp. 427–28)

DEVELOPMENTAL TRAUMA DISORDER[1]

A. Exposure

    1. Multiple or chronic exposure to one or more forms of developmentally adverse interpersonal trauma (abandonment, betrayal, physical assaults, sexual assaults, threats to bodily integrity, coercive practices, emotional abuse, witnessing violence and death).

    2. Subjective experience (rage, betrayal, fear, resignation, defeat, shame).

B. Triggered pattern of repeated dysregulation in response to trauma cues. Dysregulation (high or low) in presence of cues. Changes persist and do not return to baseline; not reduced in intensity by conscious awareness.

- Affective
- Somatic (physiological, motoric, medical)
- Behavioral (e.g., reenactment, cutting)
- Cognitive (thinking that it is happening again, confusion, dissociation, depersonalization)
- Relational (clinging, oppositional, distrustful, compliant)
- Self-attribution (self-hate and blame)

C. Persistently altered attributions and expectancies

- Negative self-attribution
- Distrust protective caretaker
- Loss of expectancy of protection by others
- Loss of trust in social agencies to protect
- Lack of recourse to social justice/retribution
- Inevitability of future victimization

D. Functional impairment

- Educational
- Family
- Peer
- Legal
- Vocational

---

1. From van der Kolk, 2005, Developmental Trauma Disorder: A New, Rational Diagnosis for Children with Complex Trauma Histories. *Psychiatric Annals,* 374–378, 401–408.

DISORDERS OF EXTREME STRESS (DESNOS)[1]

I. Alteration in Regulation of Affect and Impulses (A and 1 of B–F required):

  A. Affect Regulation (2)

  B. Modulation of Anger (2)

  C. Self-Destructive

  D. Suicidal Preoccupation

  E. Difficulty Modulating Sexual Involvement

  F. Excessive Risk-Taking

II. Alterations in Attention or Consciousness (A or B required):

  A. Amnesia

  B. Transient Dissociative Episodes and Depersonalization

III. Alterations in Self-Perception (Two of A–F required):

  A. Ineffectiveness

  B. Permanent Damage

  C. Guilt and Responsibility

  D. Shame

  E. Nobody Can Understand

  F. Minimizing

IV. Alterations in Relations With Others (One of A–C required):

  A. Inability to Trust

  B. Revictimization

  C. Victimizing Others

V. Somatization (Two of A–E required):

  A. Digestive System

  B. Chronic Pain

  C. Cardiopulmonary Symptoms

  D. Conversion Symptoms

  E. Sexual Symptoms

VI. Alterations in Systems of Meaning (A or B required):

  A. Despair and Hopelessness

  B. Loss of Previously Sustaining Beliefs

1. From Luxenberg, Spiazzola & van der Kolk (2001). *Complex Traumas and Disorders of Extreme Stress (DESNOS)*. Diagnoses, Part I: Assessment in *Directions in Psychiatry*, 21, lesson 2. Reprinted with permission.

REFERENCES

Aron, E. (1996). *The highly sensitive person.* New York: Broadway Books.

American heritage dictionary of the English language, 4th ed. (2006). Boston: Houghton Mifflin.

American Psychiatric Association. (2000). *Diagnostic and statistical manual of mental disorders*, 4th ed, text revision. Washington, DC: American Psychiatric Association.

APA Presidential Task Force on Evidence-Based Practice (May–June, 2006). Evidence-based practice in psychology. *American Psychologist, 61*, 4, 271–285.

Bergmann, U. (2008). She's come undone: A neurological exploration of dissociative disorders. In C. Forgash & M. Copeley (Eds.), *Healing the heart of trauma and dissociation with EMDR and ego state therapy.* New York: Springer.

Bernstein, E.M., & Putnam, F.W. (1986). Development, reliability, and validity of a dissociation scale. *Journal of Nervous & Mental Disease, 174*, 727–735.

Bohus, M. J., Landwehrmeyer, G. B., Stiglmayr, C. E., Limberger, M. F., Bohme, R., & Schmahl, C. G. (1999). Naltrexone in the treatment of dissociative symptoms in patients with borderline personality disorder: an open-label trial. *Journal of Clinical Psychiatry, 60*, 598–603.

Braun, B. G. (1988, March). Continuum of dissociation. *Journal of Dissociation, 1*, 1.

Brown, L. (2008). *Cultural competence in trauma therapy: Beyond the flashback.* Washington, DC: American Psychological Association.

Callahan, R., & Trubo, R. (2002). Tapping the healer within: Using thought-field therapy to instantly conquer your fears, anxieties, and emotional distress. New York: McGraw-Hill.

Chapman, A., & Gratz, K. (2007). *The borderline personality disorder survival guide.* Oakland, CA: New Harbinger.

Chertoff, J. (1998). Psychodynamic assessment and treatment of traumatized clients. *Journal of Psychotherapy Practice and Research, 7*(January), 35–46.

Cole, J. (2005). The reenactment protocol. In R. Shapiro (Ed.), *EMDR solutions: Pathways to healing* (pp. 8–56). New York: Norton.

Courtois, C. A., & Ford, J. D. (Eds.). (2009). *Treating complex post-traumatic stress disorders.* New York: Guilford.

Davanloo, H. (1980). *Short-term dynamic psychotherapy.* New York: Jason Aronson.

Davidson, J. R. T. (2004). Long-term treatment and prevention of posttraumatic stress disorder. *Journal of Clinical Psychiatry, 65,* 44–48.

Dictionary.com (2009). Trauma. Retrieved April 4, 2009, from http://dictionary.reference.com/browse/trauma/

Difede, J., Hoffman, H. G. (2002). Virtual reality exposure therapy for World Trade Center post-traumatic stress disorder: A case report. *CyberPsychology and Behavior, 5*(6), 529–535.

Doerfler, T. (2009). Non-entrainment neurofeedback. *Naturopathic Doctor News and Review, 4.* Retrieved from www.ndnr.com

Emmerson, G. (2003). *Ego state therapy.* Camathen, Wales: Crown House.

Feinstein, D. (2008). Energy psychology: A review of the preliminary evidence. *Psychotherapy: Theory, Research, Practice, Training, 45*(2), 199–213.

Foa, E. B., Hembree, E. A., & Rothbaum, B. O. (2007). Prolonged exposure therapy for PTSD: Emotional processing of traumatic experiences, therapist guide. New York: Oxford University Press.

Foa, E. B., Keane, T. M., & Friedman, M. J. (2000). *Effective treatment for PTSD.* New York: Guilford.

Foa, E. B., & Kozak, M. J. (1986). Emotional processing of fear: Exposure to corrective information. *Psychological Bulletin, 99,* 20–35.

Forgash, C., & Copeley, M. (Eds.). (2008). Healing the heart of trauma and dissociation with EMDR and ego state therapy. New York: Springer.

Fosha, D. (2000). The transforming power of affect: A model for accelerated change. New York: Basic Books.

Fraser, G. A. (2003). Fraser's "dissociative table technique" revisited, revised: A strategy for working with ego states in dissociative disorders and ego state therapy. *Dissociation, 44,* 5–28.

Freud, A. (1967). Comments on trauma: Psychic trauma. In S. Furst (Ed.), *Psychic trauma* (pp. 235–246). New York: Basic Books.

Gold, M. S., Pottash, A. C., Sweeney, D., Martin, D., & Extein, I. (1982). Antimanic, anti-depressant and antipanic effects of opiates: Clinical neuroanatomical and biochemical evidence. *Annals of the New York Academy of Sciences, 398,* 140–150.

Goleman, D. (1985). Vital lies, simple truths: The psychology of self deception. New York: Simon and Schuster.

Grand, D. (n.d.). *Brainspotting manual, phase one.* Retrieved from http://www.brainspotting.pro/

Greenwald, R. (1999). *EMDR in child and adolescent psychotherapy.* New York: Jason Aronson.

Grove, D., & Panzer, B. I. (1989). *Resolving traumatic memories.* New York: Irvington.

Hammarberg, M. (1992). Penn inventory for posttraumatic stress disorder: Psychometric properties. *Psychological Assessment, 4,* 67–76.

Hart, J., Gunnar, M., & Cicchetti, D. (1995). Salivary cortisol in maltreated children: Evidence of relations between neuroendocrine activity and social competence. *Development and Psychopathology, 7,* 11–26.

Hayes, S. C., Strosahl, K. D., & Wilson, K. G. (1999). Acceptance and commitment therapy: An experiential approach to behavior change. New York: Guilford.

Hollifield, M., Sinclair-Lian, N., Warner, T. D., & Hammerschlag, R. (2007). Acupuncture for posttraumatic stress disorder: A randomized controlled pilot trial. *Journal of Nervous and Mental Disease, 195*(6), 504–513.

Hughes, D., & Becker-Weidman, A. (2008). Dyadic developmental psychotherapy: An evidence-based treatment for children with complex trauma and disorders of attachment. *Child and Family Social Work, 13,* 329–337.

Janet, P. (1907). *The major symptoms of hysteria.* London: Macmillan.

Johnson, D. R., Hadar, L., & Ochberg, F. (2007). *The counting method (manual).* New Haven, CT: Post Traumatic Stress Center.

Junger, S. (2010). *War.* New York: Twelve.

Kabat-Zinn, J. (1990). Full catastrophe living: Using the wisdom of your body and mind to face stress, pain, and illness. New York: Dell.

Kiessling, R. (2005). Integrating resource development strategies into your EMDR practice. In R. Shapiro (Ed.), *EMDR solutions: Pathways to healing* (pp. 57–87). New York: Norton.

Kitchur, M. (2005). The strategic developmental model for EMDR. In R. Shapiro (Ed.), *EMDR solutions: Pathways to healing* (pp. 8–56). New York: Norton.

Kluft, R. P. (1988). Playing for time: Temporizing techniques in the treatment of multiple personality disorder. *American Journal of Clinical Hypnosis, 32,* 90–98.

Knipe, J. (2005). Targeting positive affect to clear the pain of unrequited love, codependence, avoidance and procrastination. In R. Shapiro (Ed.), *EMDR solutions: Pathways to healing* (pp. 189–212). New York: Norton.

Knipe, J. (2009). "Shame is my safe place": Adaptive information processing methods of resolving chronic shame-based depression. In R. Shapiro (Ed.), *EMDR solutions II: For depression, eating disorders, performance, and more* (pp. 49–89). New York: Norton.

Lambert, M. J., & Barley, D. E. (2001). Research summary on the therapeutic relationship and psychotherapy outcome. *Psychotherapy, 38*(4), 357–361.

Lanius, R. A., Williamson, P. C., Boksman, K., Densmore, M., Gupta, M.,

Neufeld, R. W., et al. (2002). Brain activation during script-driven imagery induced dissociative responses in PTSD: A functional magnetic resonance imaging investigation. *Biological Psychiatry, 52,* 305–311.

Lanius, U. F. (2002). *Trauma, neuroscience and EMDR.* Invited address, EMDRAC AGM. Vancouver, BC.

Lanius, U. F. (2003). *The neurobiology of attachment and dissociation: Clinical implications.* Invited presentation at conference, Complex Trauma Treatment Approaches, Loch Lomond Shores, Balloch, Glasgow, Scotland, October 10, 2000.

Lanius, U. F. (2005). EMDR processing with dissociative clients: Adjunctive use of opioid antagonists. In R. Shapiro (Ed.), *EMDR solutions: Pathways to healing* (pp. 121–146). New York: Norton.

Leeds, A. (2009). A guide to the standard EMDR protocols for clinicians, supervisors, and consultants. New York: Springer.

Levine, P. (1997). *Waking the tiger: Healing trauma.* Berkeley: North Atlantic Books.

Levine, S. (1991). Additional visualizations for emotional and physical pain. In *Guided meditations, explorations, and healings.* New York: Doubleday.

Linehan, M. (1993). Cognitive-behavioral treatment of borderline personality disorder. New York: Guilford.

Liotti, G. (2006). A model of dissociation based on attachment theory and research. *Journal of Trauma and Dissociation, 7*(4), 55–73.

Lovell, C. (2005). Utilizing EMDR and DBT in Trauma and Recovery Groups. In R. Shapiro (Ed.), *EMDR solutions: Pathways to healing* (pp. 263–282). New York: Norton.

Lovett, J. (1999). Small wonders: Healing childhood trauma with EMDR. New York: Free Press.

Luxenberg, T., Spinazzola, J., & van der Kolk, B. A. (2001). Complex traumas and disorders of extreme stress (DESNOS) diagnoses, Part I: Assessment. *Directions in Psychiatry, 21,* lesson 25. Retrieved April 4, 2009, from http://www.traumacenter.org/products/pdf_files/DESNOS.pdf

Ma, M. (2009, May 17) Prescription for vets: Meditation. *Seattle Times.*

Main, M. (1991). Metacognitive knowledge, metacognitive monitoring and singular (coherent) versus multiple (incoherent) models of attachment: Findings and directions for further research. In C. Parkes, J. Stevenson-Hinde, & P. Marris (Eds.), *Attachment across the life cycle* (pp. 127–159). London: Routledge.

Malan, D. H. (1976). *The frontier of brief psychotherapy.* New York: Plenum.

Manfield, P. (Ed.). (1998). *Extending EMDR.* New York: Norton.

McFarlane, A. C., Yehuda, R. (1996). Resilience, vulnerability and the course of posttraumatic reactions. In B. A. van der Kolk, A. C. McFarlane, & L. Weisaeth (Eds.), *Traumatic stress: The effects of overwhelming experience on mind, body and society* (pp. 155–181). New York: Guilford.

McGoldrick, M., & Gerson, R. (1985). *Genograms in family assessment.* New York: Norton.

McGoldrick, M., & Gerson, R. (1999). *Genograms: Assessment and Intervention.* New York: Norton.

Meichenbaum, D. (1996). Stress inoculation for coping with stressors. *Clinical Psychologist, 49,* 4–7.

Menahemi, A., & Ariel, E. (1997). *Doing time, doing Vipassana.* Karuna Films.

Neborsky, R. (2006). A clinical model for the comprehensive treatment of trauma using an affect-experiencing-attachment theory approach. In M. F. Solomon & D. J. Siegel (Eds.), *Healing trauma* (pp. 282–321). New York: Norton.

Ochberg, F. (1996). The counting method. *Journal of Traumatic Stress, 9,* 887–894.

Ogden P., Minton, K., & Pain, C. (2006). Trauma and the body: A sensorimotor approach to psychotherapy. New York: Norton.

O'Shea, K. (2009). The EMDR early trauma protocol. In R. Shapiro (Ed.), *EMDR solutions II: For depression, eating disorders, performance, and more* (pp. 313–334. New York: Norton.

Pace, P. (2007). *Lifespan integration: Connecting ego-states through time.* Self-published. Retrieved from http://www.lifespanintegration.com/book.php

Panksepp, J. (1998). Affective neuroscience: The foundations of human and animal emotions. New York: Oxford University Press.

Paulsen, S. (2009). Looking through the eyes of trauma and dissociation: An illustrated guide for EMDR therapists and clients. Bainbridge Island, WA: Bainbridge Institute for Integrative Psychology.

Paulsen, S., & Lanius, U. (2009). Toward an embodied self: Integrating EMDR with somatic and ego state interventions. In R. Shapiro (Ed.), *EMDR solutions II: For depression, eating disorders, performance, and more* (pp. 335–388). New York: Norton.

Peniston, E. G., & Kulkosky, P. J. (1991). Alpha-theta brainwave neurofeedback therapy for Vietnam veterans with combat-related posttraumatic stress disorder. *Medical Psychotherapy: An International Journal, 4,* 47–60.

Peniston, E. G., & Kulkosky, P. J. (1992). Alpha-theta EEG biofeedback training in alcoholism and posttraumatic stress disorder. *International Society for the Study of Subtle Energies and Energy Medicines, 2,* 5–7.

Perry, B. D. (2000). *Traumatized children: How childhood trauma influences brain development.* Retrieved October 17, 2001, from www.childtrauma.org/ctamate rials/trau_cami.asp

Phillips, P., & Stein, A. M. (2008). *The Dhamma Brothers.* Freedom Behind Bars Productions. Retrieved from http://www.dhammabrothers.com/

Porges, S. W. (1995). Orienting in a defensive world. *Psychophysiology, 32*(4), 301–318.

Porges, S. W. (2001). The oolyvagal theory: Phylogenetic substrates of a social nervous system. *Physiology and Behavior, 79,* 503–513.

Porges, S. W. (2005). The role of social engagement in attachment and bonding, a phylogenetic perspective. In C. S. Carter, L. Ahnert, K. E. Grossmann, S. B. Hardy, M. E. Lamb, S. W. Porges, & N. Sachser (Eds.), *Attachment and bonding: A new synthesis* (pp. 33–54). Cambridge, MA: MIT Press.

Raskind, M. A., Peskind, E. R., Kanter, E. D., Petrie, E. C., Radant, A., Thompson, C. E., et al. (2003, February). Reduction of nightmares and other PTSD symptoms in combat veterans by prazosin: A placebo-controlled study. *American Journal of Psychiatry, 160*, 371–373.

Resick, P. A., & Schnicke, M. K. (1992). Cognitive processing therapy for sexual assault victims. *Journal of Consulting and Clinical Psychology, 60*(5), 748–756.

Resick, P. A., & Schnicke, M. K. (1993). Cognitive processing therapy for rape victims: A treatment manual. Newbury Park, CA: Sage.

Ross, C. A. (1997). Dissociative identity disorder: Diagnosis, clinical features, and treatment of multiple personality, 2nd ed. New York: John Wiley & Sons.

Rothbaum, B. O., Hodges, L., Alarcon, R., Ready, D., Shahar, F., Graap, K., et al. (1999). Virtual reality exposure therapy for PTSD vietnam veterans: A case study. *Journal of Traumatic Stress, 12*(2), 263–271.

Rothbaum, B. O., Meadows, E. A., Resick, P., & Foy, D. W. (2000). "Cognitive-behavioral therapy." In E. B. Foa, T. M. Keane, & M. J. Friedman (Eds.), *Effective treatment for PTSD.* New York: Guilford.

Schiraldi, G. R. (2000). *The post-traumatic stress disorder sourcebook.* Lincolnwood, IL: Lowell House.

Schmahl, C., Stiglmayr, C., Böhme, R., & Bohus, M. (1999). [Treatment of dissociative symptoms in borderline patients with naltrexone] (in German). *Nervenarzt, 70*, 262–264.

Schmidt, S. J. (2009). The developmental needs meeting strategy: A model for healing adults with childhood attachment wounds. San Antonio, TX: DNMS Institute.

Schore, A. N. (1994). Affect regulation and the origin of the self: The neurobiology of emotional development. Hillsdale, NJ: Erlbaum.

Schore, A. N. (2009). *Working in the right brain: A regulation model of clinical expertise for treatment of attachment trauma.* Paper presented at Current Approaches to Treatment of Trauma Conference, Lifespan Learning Center, UCLA, March 29, 2009.

Schwartz, L. (2008). *Brainspotting II Class.* Whidbey Island, Washington.

Schwartz, R. (1995). *Internal family systems therapy.* New York: Guilford.

Scott, C., & Briere, J. (2006). Biology and psychopharmacology of trauma. In J. Briere & C. Scott (Eds.), *Principles of trauma therapy: A guide to symptoms, evaluation, and treatment* (pp. 185–230). Thousand Oaks, CA: Sage.

Shapiro, F. (2001). Eye movement desensitization and reprocessing: Basic principles, protocols and procedures (2nd ed.). New York: Guilford.

Shapiro, R. (2005). The two-hand interweave. In R. Shapiro (Ed.), *EMDR solutions: Pathways to healing* (pp. 160–188). New York: Norton.

Shapiro, R. (2009a). Attachment-based depression: Healing the hunkered down. In R. Shapiro (Ed.), *EMDR solutions II: For depression, eating disorders, performance, and more* (pp. 90–106). New York: Norton.

Shapiro, R. (2009b). Endogenous depression and mood disorders. In R. Shapiro (Ed.), *EMDR solutions II: For depression, eating disorders, performance, and more* (pp. 24–48). New York: Norton.

Shipherd, J. C., Street, A. E., & Resick, P. A. (2006). Cognitive therapy for post-traumatic stress disorder. In V. M. Follette & J. I. Ruzek (Eds.), *Cognitive-Behavioral Therapies for Trauma* (pp. 96–116). New York: Guilford.

Siegel, D. J. (1999). The developing mind: Toward a neurobiology of interpersonal experience. New York: Guilford.

Siegel, D. J. (2003). Q & A at New Developments in Attachment Theory: Applications to Clinical Practice, UCLA, Los Angeles, March 8.

Siegel, D. J. (2007). The mindful brain: Reflection and attunement in the cultivation of well-being. New York: Norton.

Siegel, D. J. (2009, March). *A systems view of disintegration and integration.* Presentation at the UCLA Lifespan Learning Trauma Conference, Los Angeles.

Silver, S. (2009). EMDR and the Treatment of War and Terrorism Survivors: Working with the Latest Generation. Workshop in Olympia, WA, November 7 and 8.

Silver, S., & Rogers, S. (2002). Light in the heart of darkness: EMDR and the treatment of war and terrorism survivors. New York: Norton.

Steele, A. (2007). *Developing a secure self: An attachment-based approach to adult psychotherapy* (2nd ed.). Gabriola, BC: Author. Retrieved from http://www.april-steele.ca/

Steele, K., van der Hart, O., & Nijenhuis, E. (2005). Phase-oriented treatment of structural dissociation in complex traumatization: Overcoming trauma-related phobias. *Journal of Trauma and Dissociation, 6*(3).

Stein, J. (2008). Letters from the Dhamma Brothers: Meditation behind bars. Onalaska, WA: Pariyatti Press.

Stickgold, R. (2001). *A putative neurobiological mechanism of action.* Plenary at EMDRIA Conference, Austin, TX.

Taylor, F., & Raskind, M. A. (2002). The alpha1-adrenergic antagonist prazosin improves sleep and nightmares in civilian trauma posttraumatic stress disorder. *Journal of Clinical Psychopharmacology, 22*(1), 82–85.

Tronick, E. (2007). The neurobehavioral and social-emotional development of infants and children. New York: Norton.

Tull, M. (2009). Stress inoculation training. Retrieved November 10, 2009, from http://ptsd.about.com/od/glossary/g/SIT_Def.htm

Turner, E. (2005). Affect regulation for children through art, play, and storytelling. In R. Shapiro (Ed.), *EMDR solutions: Pathways to healing* (pp. 327–344). New York: Norton.

Twombly, J. (2005). EMDR for clients with DID, DDNOS, and ego states. In R.

Shapiro (Ed.), *EMDR solutions: Pathways to healing* (pp. 88–120). New York: Norton.

Twombly, J., & Schwartz, R. (2008). The integration of the internal family systems model and EMDR. In C. Forgash & M. Copeley (Eds.), *Healing the heart of trauma and dissociation with EMDR and ego state therapy*. New York: Springer.

van der Hart, O., Nijenhuis, E., & Steele, K. (2006). The haunted self: Structural dissociation and the treatment of chronic traumatization. New York: Norton.

van der Kolk, B. A. (1996). Traumatic stress: The effects of overwhelming experience on mind, body, and society. New York: Guilford.

van der Kolk, B. A. (2005). Developmental trauma disorder: A new, rational diagnosis for children with complex trauma histories. *Psychiatric Annals, 374–378, 401–408*. Retrieved April 4, 2009, from http://www.traumacenter.org/products/pdf_files/Preprint_Dev_Trauma_Disorder.pdf

van der Kolk, B. A. (2006). Clinical implications of neuroscience research in PTSD. *Annals of the New York Academy of Sciences 1071, 277–293*.

van der Kolk, B. A., Spinazzola, J., Blaustein, M. E., Hopper, J. W., Hopper, E. K., Korn, D. L., et al.. (2007). A randomized clinical trial of eye movement desensitization and reprocessing (EMDR), fluoxetine, and pill placebo in the treatment of posttraumatic stress disorder: Treatment effects and long-term maintenance. *Journal of Clinical Psychiatry, 68*(1), 37–46.

Walser, R. D., & Hayes, S. C. (2006). Acceptance and commitment therapy in the treatment of posttraumatic stress disorder. In V. M. Follette & R. I. Ruzek (Eds.), *Cognitive-behavioral therapies for trauma*. New York: Guilford.

Walser, R. D., & Westrup, D. (2007). Acceptance and commitment therapy for the treatment of post-traumatic stress disorders and trauma related problems. Oakland, CA: New Harbinger.

Wills, D. K. (2007, June). Heal life's traumas. *Yoga Journal*. Retrieved May 30, 2009, from www.yogajournal.com/health/2532

Wilson, S., & Tinker, R. (2005). The phantom limb pain protocol. In R. Shapiro (Ed.), *EMDR solutions: Pathways to healing* (pp. 147–159). New York: Norton.

Wolpe, J. (1958). *Psychotherapy by reciprocal inhibition*. Stanford, CA: Stanford University Press.

Index